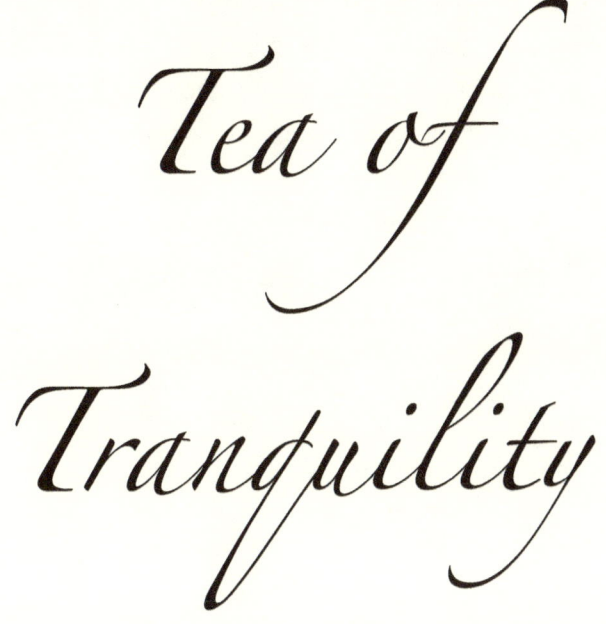

Tea of Tranquility

Making herbal teas that support tranquility and
nervous system function

By: Brooke E. Criswell

Bewell Bohemia
Herbs and Things

Copyright

Reclaimer (reclaiming individual autonomy for wellness)

The content of this book is for educational use only, providing helpful information on the subjects discussed. No discussion serves as medical advice. While the information included is well-researched and presented with care, I, Brooke Criswell, am trained herbalists and not licensed or registered healthcare practitioner. You are responsible for your own well being. You must consider what you know of your body and make your decisions with support of a wellness team (including medical professionals) that you trust and respect. This book offers information for your consideration. You are responsible for all decisions regarding your wellness, whether you read the information in a book, on the internet, hear it from a friend, family member, or medical professional. Please consult your medical care provider before using herb recipe or recommendation, particularly if you have a known medical condition or if you are pregnant or nursing. Some herbs are contraindicated with certain pharmaceutical drugs. People are complex and individual, and as such may interact with an herb differently than other people.

References are provided for informational purposes only and do not constitute endorsement of any websites or other sources. Readers should be aware that the websites listed in this book may change.

Dedication

Thanks to the Otterbein Public Library, where the "Tea of Tranquility" workshop was initially held, and to the ladies who attended the preceding workshop, "Through Thyme and Space."

Table of Contents

Introduction

Tea of Tranquility, a name inspired by the Sea of Tranquility, as the workshop, held on the 50th anniversary of the lunar landing, celebrated the moon, a sense of exploration and a quest for tranquility. The workshop was first offered at a public library during a summer of programs themed "A Universe of Stories." I wanted the workshops I led to link with the theme; hence, "Tea of Tranquility."

Below I include a quote from the NASA website in which a description of the experience of lunar landing is shared.

""Magnificent desolation," said Aldrin.

Those two words summed up the yin-yang of the Moon. The impact craters, the toppled boulders, the layers of moondust-it was utterly alien. Yet Tranquillity Base felt curiously familiar, like home. Later Apollo astronauts had similar feelings. Maybe this comes from staring at the Moon so often from Earth. Or maybe it's because the Moon is a piece of Earth, spun off our young planet billions of years ago. No one knows; it just is."

from "Wide Awake on the Sea of Tranquility," a post on the NASA website.[1] 50 years ago astronauts with the aid of their vast support team, succeeded at landing on the moon, that most familiar and mysterious celestial object. What aspirations fuel your dreams? What unsung support team fosters your success?

"Tea of Tranquility" is a hands-on workshop of exploration. Participants craft an individually selected tea blend to lift mood,

---

[1]Dunbar, Brian. "Wide Awake on the Sea of Tranquillity." *NASA*, NASA, 16 Mar. 2015, www.nasa.gov/exploration/home/19jul_seaoftranquillity.html.

soothe mind, calm nerves; in other words, support tranquility through a connection with the nervous system.

The nervous system, that electric wonder, that control system of our bodies - sending and receiving signals, like astronauts and ground control; activating and ceasing processes based on need, interpreting the world outside (and inside) our lunar shuttle of self. Here is to a sense of exploration, here is to the moon, that celestial wonder, and here is to tranquility.

Hi! Brooke here, with a brief introduction to me. I love plants, down to my very roots. Always have. Maybe it is born of my childhood spent exploring the woods of western Pennsylvania, outside all day in summer, and most evenings after school fall, winter, and spring. I loved to munch on wild onions in spring, and chase falling leaves in autumn. Even today the scent of crumbled sycamore or tulip tree leaves inspires joy.

My passion for plants guided me into herbalism. I am a budding herbalist. On my quest to learn about plants and their many and varied relationships with people, I do much reading and researching. I attended various programs and completed courses in herbal study, beginning with an introductory course "Roots of Herbalism" through the Florida School of Holistic Living. I then progressed to a comprehensive program through Chestnut School of Herbal Medicine entitled "Herbal Immersion." Herbalist pursue an ongoing education journey, and thus, in addition to the above listed programs I have attended various webinars offered through the American Herbalist Guild, and other herbal study programs. I am now enrolled in courses offered by Commonwealth Center of Holistic Herbalism.

Simultaneous to study, I started a cottage business, BeWell Bohemia Herbs and Things, in which I propagate plants from seed or cutting and sell them at local garden expos and farmers markets.

I wanted folks who bought my plants to have some insight into not only the growing conditions favored by that plant, but also into its herbal medicinal aspects. So, I sat down, gathered my research, personal observations, and garden journals to craft an herbal monograph for each plant I sell. This book includes featured herbs from that collection of monographs. May you enjoy turning (or scrolling) the pages. Here's to healthy relationships with plants and personal wellness.

Brooke E. Criswell

BeWell Bohemia Herbs and Things

bewellbohemia@gmail.com

Wellness,

a many-faceted concept

Before I introduce the featured herbs of the worksop and recipes, let me talk about wellness in general. I am not a medical professional. I do not offer medical advice, nothing in the book is medical advice.

What I offer is discussion about individual responsibility for personal wellness. As an Herbalist, I study, observe, and explore herbs. Herbs support our wellness in many and varied ways; through the actions of phytochemical constituents, through plant/person relationships, and through ritual, for example the ritual of making tea. However, herbs are only one facet of a journey to wellness, if we don't look at the other aspects of our lifestyle, we will not develop and support wellness. Movement, nourishment, interconnection (community, spirituality), emotion, mental stimulation, rest… are all essential facets of wellness.

This text is not dedicated to a deep discussion of the above facets of wellness. I do encourage you to reflect on your lifestyle. Are your choices supporting your wellness? Are you nourishing your mind-body-spirit? Are you moving often enough to support physical wellness? Are you finding laughter and joy in your life? Are your setting aside sufficient time for rest? Are you balancing your obligations to prevent overload?

Tranquility involves managing stress, eating nourishing food, getting abundant rest, engaging in meaningful spiritual practice, connecting socially in supportive communities, stimulating your mind, moving (being physically active), and attending to self-care.

Tranquility is a process as much as it is a product.

Tranquility is connected to peace of mind, restful spirit, relaxed body, and more, depending on your perspective. What is your idea of tranquility? What do you envision as peace of mind-body-spirit? How is your tranquility created? Supported? Close your eyes and imagine yourself tranquil? Try to note what that feels like, emotionally and physically? What is it like internally and externally?

If that sounds like too many questions to tackle, don't consider them all at once. Choose one. Think on it. Maybe journal or find a way of expressing your thoughts. Then choose one action that supports your wellness. You do not have to manage everything. At once.

As you add herbal tea into your quest for tranquility, attend to the ritual of making tea. The pause to select and prepare tea, the sequences of preparing the teapot and cup, the warmth and aroma of the steeping tea and the feel of the cup in your hand. For extra tranquility, select a cup that brings.you peace or makes you smile. Choose a favorite from your cupboard, or splurge on a new cup. Check the thrift shops, which boast a bounty of cups from whimsical to formal. In fact, consider choosing a tea set or stemware that is satisfying and inspiring to you. If you are making tea regularly, then surely the frequent use of an item justifies having stemware of quality. Perhaps the mason jar you use symbolizes your grandmother putting up summer produce. Maybe the french/press reminds you of college days or a trip to a city. Maybe the teapot makes you feel like you are at Downton Abby. Maybe the weight or shape of the jar, glass, mug, press, or teapot, feels 'just right'. Maybe the motif or print is of your favorite flower, or animal, or in some way brings you joy. Whatever the connection, choose steep-ware for yourself. Each step of the process can build tranquility.

I know that when I garden, I am being active. I am moving lots of different muscles in lots of different ways. Gardening involves stretching to reach, lifting objects of various weights, some heavy to me. I stand, sit, squat, bend, walk. All of this movement fuels my physical wellness. I have a low capacity for exertion without pain, so I am thrilled how much activity I get while gardening. I move at my own pace, sometimes slowly, nonetheless, I move! While I am gardening I am also outside, my skin absorbing sunlight and making precious vitamin D. My eyes recording the natural light, and noting daily rhythms, which drive my circadian rhythms. By being in natural light in the morning, I trigger stimulation of hormones, and support the daily rhythm of cortisol that will foster quality sleep. The activity also helps foster sleep. Gardening also helps me mitigate stress and elevate mood. I feel relaxed during and after gardening. Gardening also affords me time in nature, which is well recognized as an important aspect of human wellness. The sky, the sun, the clouds, the trees, the leaves, the flowers, the insects, the birds, and even the fresh air all contribute to my emotional, mental, and spiritual well/being.

I talk so much about gardening because it exemplifies many facets of wellness. Ways gardening supports my tranquility: is fun, supports physical well/being in many ways from chemical to skeletal muscular, and everything in between, lifts mood, provides spiritual connection, yields herbs for tea of tranquility. Many facets of wellness intricately interconnected.

I encourage you to support your tranquility, which also supports your overall wellness, one action (or inaction) at a time. You can. Even small actions, quiet choices, little moments are effective.

BeWell.

You deserve it.

Yardening

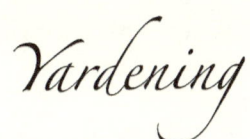

Yes I meant yardening, it is not a typographical error. I will refer to the yarden, and yardening in the book, so I wanted to include an introduction to the term.

My approach to gardening encompasses a philosophy of "yard as garden; garden as yard," My philosophy involves assessing the various habitats of the property, observing what is already growing there, then using permaculture principles to create yarden that requires the least work input for the highest function output. I have a grassy plot under the clothesline, I herb beds along the house border, I have raised beds, vegetable plots and a compost pile. I also have patches of volunteer plant communities, that succeed each other seasonally. Early spring violets, followed by columbine (and the attending hummingbirds), which transitions to larkspur, eventually shaded by the mature poke towering at six feet. The cycle of constant blooms provides consistent food for pollinators, and resources for me and myhousehold. From food, to medicine, to aesthetic beauty, we are nourished by our yardens.

I work in time with the seasons, and plant plants suited to each respective niche. Spring sees me excitingly gathering violets, summer harvesting squash, and fall digging dandelion root.

I grow vegetables and flowers, like many gardeners. I also embrace the tenacious plants, often called weeds, such as dandelion, plantain, ground ivy, and the like, as welcome member to the yarden community. I support biodiversity, I compost, and I tend to plants. I also let plants have their way a bit, which may make my yarden look untended, or wild. It is wild, in that much wildlife can be found. I thrill to the daily bird activity, the buzz of pollinator, the chatter of squirrel and chipmunk, and the presence of a few rabbits. The balance of the biodiversity makes a healthy and productive yarden.

Herbalism

You do not need to have an understanding of herbalism to use this book. The recipes do not rely on your mastery of terms or concepts associated with herbalism. The garden information in the monographs is useful regardless of your herbalism affinity. If you are curious or want to know a bit about herbalism, then I include this brief discussion for you.

Herbalism is the use of plants to support wellness.

Herbalism is a vast and diverse field, so this introduction is neither comprehensive nor definitive. Depending on your focus, philosophy, and intention, the aspects of herbalism vary widely. The herbalist community embraces such diversity. Herbalism includes folks who grow the plants, harvest the plants, prepare herbal concoctions, study the plants, conduct clinical visits. Herbalists are botanists, gardeners, business owners, teachers, care givers, and so much more. The American Herbalist Guild, states, on their website, "Herbalists are people who dedicate their lives to working with medicinal plants. They include native healers, scientists, naturopaths, holistic medical doctors, researchers, writers, herbal pharmacists, medicine makers, wild crafters, harvesters, and herbal farmers to name a few. While herbalists are quite varied, the common love and respect for life, especially the relationship between plants and humans, unites them. Persons specializing in the therapeutic use of plants may be medical herbalists, traditional herbalists, acupuncturists, midwives, naturopathic physicians, or even one's own grandmother." [2] The American Herbalist Guild's (AHG) primary goal is to promote a high level of professionalism and education in the study and practice of therapeutic herbalism."[3] The AHG website is an excellent source if you would like to learn more about herbalism.

Herbalism possess a long history, with cultures across the globe developing in relation to the plants surrounding that respective community, and changing with the times. You can look to Ayurveda, Chinese, German, or "Western" herbalism traditions to see what I mean.

Herbalism is an approach to wellness that incorporates plants, as food and medicine, sometimes as spiritual influence. Herbalism, in its conception of wellness, recognizes the context of the individual's lifestyle as part of the pursuit of wellness and balance. As such, herbalism encompasses much more than which phytochemical interact with which body system in which way. Herbalism does not follow a "if you have a sore throat, then blank herb will help" approach. Much more than a symptom is involved in the discussion of wellness and plants to support wellness. Herbalism is a discipline that strives to look beyond the symptom into the source of imbalance and the internal and external factors that influence balance, or imbalance. That is to say, herbalism is holistic. Herbalism is synergistic: the sum is more the the parts.

I view herbalism as fostering relationships with plants. But, that sentence might seem vague or … granola-crunchy for some. I will try to ground and flesh out the idea. Plants are the basis of

---

[2] Admin. Herbal Medicine Fundamentals. *American Herbalists Guild*, 13 Nov. 2016, www.americanherbalistsguild.com/herbal-medicine-fundamentals.

[3] American Herbalists Guild. *American Herbalists Guild*, www.americanherbalistsguild.com/.

life here on earth. Plants turn sunlight into useable food and generate breathable air, so we all rely on relationships with plants, regardless of whether we think of the interactions as 'relationships' or not. Herbalism acknowledges and celebrates these interrelationships with plants.

As an herbalist I study plants - botany, propagation, properties, phytochemistry, the minutia and the grand. Fascination with how plants function, grow, and interact inspires my study. Herbalism is about the interrelationships between plants and people, so I also study nutrition, anatomy and physiology, various dis-eases and other aspects of wellness. I strive to understand how the chemistry of the plants interacts with human chemistry. I explore how various plants, prepared in various ways, influence tissue and systems. I note Ways wellness is supported or enhanced through plants. For me, herbalism is a blend of science, observation, curiosity, and mysticism.

Holistic herbalism includes considering the person, situation, and lifestyle before determining which plants are suited to supporting wellness.

Consideration of the person involves the concept of energetics. Energetics refers to the observable way an herb impacts a person. There are three continuums along which energetics fall: hot / cold, wet / dry, and tense / lax. Tissue states fall along the conntinuums. For example, if a person has a fever they are hot. If a person has a head cold with a runny nose, the tissue is wet. So, when a plant influences a body system, the impact is often discussed in terms of energetics. For example, cayenne increases blood flow and is described as 'hot' energetically. A person's constitution, which follows the same concepts, is the way they generally tend to be. You know folks with high metabolisms, and those with a low metabolisms. You know folks that are sensitive and emotionally responsive to subtle stimuli, and others who are even-keeled and more emotionally resistant to stimuli. You know folks who tend to be warm, regardless of the surrounding temperature, and other folks who tend to be cold. These are all example of constitution. So, if an herbalist is choosing a plant to recommend to an individual, the herbalist will discuss the person's tendencies to determine likely constitution.

While constitution refers to a generally tendency, tissue state refers to fluctuating conditions in reaction to environment, ailment, or other stimuli.

An herbalist will consider the person's constitution, tissue state, and energetics of an herb to determine which herbs will support wellness most aptly.

Herbalism, a holistic approach to wellness that considers many relevant variables when matching plant to person. Herbalism, a holistic approach to wellness that celebrates human interrelationships with plants. Herbalism, a holistic discipline that incorporates an array of interests from botany to physiology.

Tea of Tranquility Featured Herbs

Catnip

Chamomile

Lavender

Lemon Balm

Tulsi

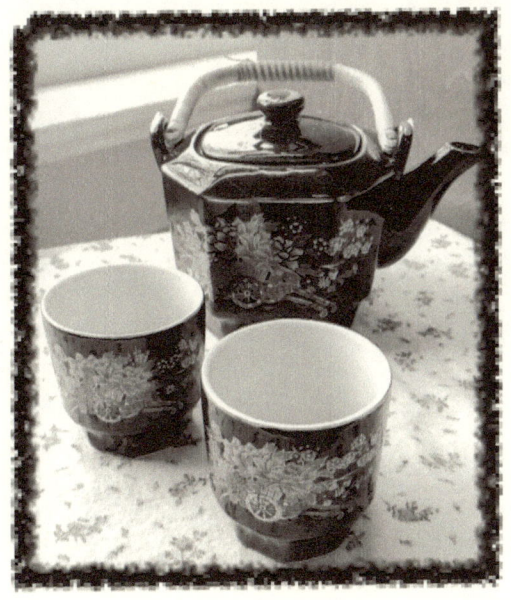

A series of herbal monographs of the above featured herbs follows.
Each monograph provides an overview of the herb, specifics for growing the herb, and a discussion of herbal uses. Enjoy.

Catnip
Nepeta cataria

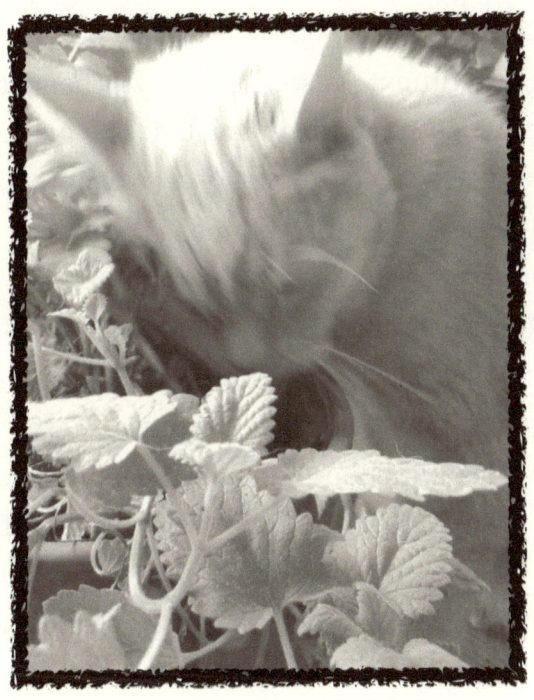

While many folks are familiar with catnip as a cat's treat, they may not be aware of its relationship with humans. I have long loved the scent and flavor of catnip tea, and value its benefits on the nervous system. Catnip is rich in a variety of constituents, which have been researched.

According to the Pharmacognosy of Nepeta Cataria, an academic article investigating the scientific composition of catnip, published in 1995, "leaves and flowering tops, which contain tannin and volatile oils are aromatic, carminative, tonic, diaphoretic, refrigerant, emmenagogue, antiseptic, and stimulant; leaves are sometimes chewed to relieve a toothache."[4] While many of those terms may be unfamiliar to you, it does show the many and varied effects catnip compounds have on people. If you want a quick definition, check the glossary in the back of the book. Know that the synergy of the many and various plant constituents, also called phytochemicals, are greater than any one constituent isolated. The plant produces the chemicals to serve its own purposes, we, humans, often benefit from the result. Catnips aroma is distinct. In fact, cats reaction to catnip is based on scent. Aromatherapy. The aromatics also are extracted in tea. Carminative refers to catnip supporting the digestive system, specifically by preventing or eliminating gas and the associated pressure. Catnip serves as a tonic because it is mild enough to be ingested daily over a long term. Catnip, therefore, can support nervous, digestive, urinary systems, and wellness overall. I have catnip in my daily morning tea blend, comprised of jasmine, catnip and lavender. A study conducted in 2017 published in the article, <u>Sustainable Manufacture of Insect Repellents derived from Nepeta cataria</u>, showed effective results. [5] Catnip as insect repellent, what a non-toxic idea.

Maybe you are not interested in all this scientific journal stuff, and prefer I just share what I have learned, so I shall share. Catnip relaxes the nervous system and promotes calm, alleviates

---

[4]Sarkar, M. et al. "Pharmacognosy of Nepeta Cataria." *Ancient Science of Life*, vol XIV, April 1995, pages 225-234.

[5]Patience, Gregory S., et al. "Sustainable Manufacture of Insect Repellents Derived from Nepeta Cataria." *Scientific Reports*, vol. 8, no. 1, 2018, doi:10.1038/s41598-017-18141-z.

anxiety, ameliorates restlessness, and supports positive mood. The effect is mild and gentle enough for children and elders. Catnip makes a great friend to chamomile, another gentle, yet deeply effective, herb.

Catnip, though too humble to boast, holds a long history of use by many cultures. Mountain Rose Herbs, a reputable and socially conscious source for herbs, asserts on their website, "Catnip was part of American folk medicine and Native American healing systems, and employed as a gentle tea for children in cases of occasional upset stomach or sleeplessness. Catnip was used by the Hoh, Delaware, and Iroquois tribes for children's complaints due to its mild nature. The Cherokee used the plant similarly to other indigenous groups and also considered it to be an overall strengthening tonic. They chose this herb when a relaxant was needed in cases of irritability or sleeplessness, just like the Europeans."[6]

In addition to excellent interactions with the nervous system, catnip impacts the digestive system by calming upset tummy, lessening the upward fire feeling associated with indigestion or heartburn sensation. That carminative action of preventing or alleviating gas in the digestive tract plays a role.

Catnip also facilitates perspiration, thereby having a cooling effect and helping the body handle a fever.[7]

Catnip is a welcome and generous friend, offering aid to many body systems. Spend some time near a patch of catnip, take in

---

[6]"Mountain Rose Herbs: Catnip." – *Mountain Rose Herbs*, www.mountainroseherbs.com/products/catnip/profile.

[7]Wells, Katie. "Benefits of Catnip & How to Use It | Wellness Mama." *Wellness Mama®*, 23 Jan. 2019, wellnessmama.com/4525/catnip-herb-profile/.

the soft fuzzy leaves, delicate blooms, and pleasant scent, and you too may love the friendly plant.

Grow, tend, and garden befriend

Access the many traits of catnip by growing it in your own garden. Catnip is easy to grow showing the same assertiveness in the garden as many other members of the mint family. Not shy to spread, you may find it best controlled in a container or raised bed. Or, plant it and await its abundant generosity. Catnip is a member of the mint family (Lamiaceae), and shares many of their common traits. Stems are square, its aromatic properties deter mosquitos, yet attract beneficial insects. Catnip grows assertively, like many mints, and will unabashed spread, so if you want to keep it contained, edge the bed well or plant it in a container. Container planted catnip, though, may not survive the winter.

Growing Conditions
Grows as an herbaceous perennial (top growth dies back, roots remain alive) in zones 3 to 8

Catnip prefers:
Moderately rich, loamy to sandy, well-draining soil
Full sun
Tolerates partial shade
pH range 6.3 to 7.3
Drought tolerant

Plant size and spacing
1 to 3 feet tall
1 foot wide, loosely bushy to lanky in character

Companion Planting Affiliations: Catnip is an herb noted for repelling certain garden pests, and therefore an ally to other plants.[8]

Pests repelled by catnip:
Aphids
Colorado potato beetle
Cucumber beetle
Flea beetle
Japanese beetle
Squash bug

Due to its growth habit, catnip may also attract beneficial insects who like "dark, cool, moist spots." Explains Rodale's Illustrated Encyclopedia of Herbs. Creating a habitat for beneficial insects supports a healthy garden. If you are using organic or sustainable gardening practices, the more biologically diverse the yarden (yard as garden, garden as yard) the less care you will need to take of it, and the more the yarden plants with thrive. I am a low-key gardener, I like to let the yarden take care of itself as much as possible.

Care notes: Water catnip regularly, especially until established; however, be sure not to over water. Allow soil to dry slightly between watering. Once the plant is established in the ground, roots strong, watering should only be necessary during long spells of dryness.

If catnip is in a container, the plant will require regular watering, and occasional feeding, since containers dry out more quickly

---

[8]Kowalchik, Claire, et al. *Rodale's Illustrated Encyclopedia of Herbs.* Rodale Press, 1987.

than the ground, and the nutrients get used up without a larger soil ecosystem to restore them. If you have a container of catnip and you have cats, the cats are likely to get into the container. Mine climbed right inside a terra cotta pot of catnip I had. The broke the branches in their ecstasy to rub in it and eat it. Poor wee catnip plant, happy happy cats.

Ways the plants support wellness

Now that your catnip is growing well, and you are ready to harvest and partake of the bounty, lets look at how and when to harvest, what the energetics and actions of catnip are, and explore some recipes.

Energetics: Warming and Cooling
If you think that sounds paradoxical, think of energetics as a way of observing how the plant impact can be sensed by the body. Sometimes the sensation varies over time, or responds differently in different tissue or systems.

Actions: antispasmodic, diaphoretic, carminative, anxiolytic, digestive stimulant

As a nervine: The manner in which catnip supports the digestive system actually often serves to support the nervous system too. Ryn Midura, of CommonWealth Center for Holistic Herbalism writes on their blog, "[Catnip is] very effective for anxiety or nervousness when its source lies in poor digestive function – when your bellyache makes you anxious. This is really common! Many, many people are walking around feeling generally ill-at-ease, only because they're not digesting their food well. The truth is, the "rest-and-digest" state is one you can get at from either end: while we usually say you've got to settle down to have happy guts, it's equally true that if you help yourself digest, you'll be better able to rest." But that is not all Ryn has to say about the nervous system interactions with catnip, "Catnip can be helpful for panic and anxiety in adults and children, including when everyone's worried together. A soothing herb, catnip is a nice nervine to take before bedtime, for times when falling asleep is difficult. Pairing it with passionflower or wood betony makes sense for either of these purposes."[9]

Parts Used: Leaves, stems, and flowers are used medicinally

When to Harvest: Gather leaves, stems, and flowers before the seeds begin to develop. Catnip, though not especially noted for its flowers, blooms from late spring to midsummer. Paying attention to bloom can inform when the plant is to be harvested. The leaves and stems can be harvested at any time, often multiple times a season. If the catnip plant is cut back (harvested) after the initial flowering, the plant may bush out and yield another harvest later in the growing season.

---

[9]Midura, Ryn. "Catnip: Herb of the Week · CommonWealth Center for Holistic Herbalism." *CommonWealth Center for Holistic Herbalism*, 17 July 2018, commonwealthherbs.com/catnip-herb-of-the-week/.

How to Prepare

When using fresh, or freshly dried, catnip, you can make a variety of herbal preparations. Even just crushing the leaves and smelling the scent. I enjoy the scent of catnip, it brings a smile to my heart. When I give it to my cats, I take a moment to smell the crushed leaves. The cats get very excited by the scent to.

Make an excellent tea - from either fresh or dried catnip
When you make tea with herb leaves or flowers, if you use fresh you will always need more plant material to get the flavor and medicinal constituents, because fresh plant leaf and bloom are comprised of mostly water. Dried herb is much more concentrated, so less plant material yields the same or greater flavor and medicinal constituent content.

To make the tea:

1. Heat the water. I like my tea piping hot, so I use water a a rolling boil, others prefer to use water that is just about to boil. Trust your preference.

2. While the water boils, prepare your steep ware. There are many ways you can make loose leaf tea. You can use a ceramic or porcelain teapot, you can use a glass French press, you can use a tea ball, or you can use a cloth teabag…. Find a system that is comfortable for you.

3. Place 2 tsp of fresh chamomile flowers or 1 tsp of dried catnip leaves per 8 oz water into teapot, press, thermos, or mason jar

4. Pour boiling water over the catnip in the steep-ware.

5. Cover! This is very important, for if uncovered the constituents will rise with the steam, and you will have a less flavorful, less potent cup of tea. If your chosen steep-ware has a lid, like a tea pot or French press, then this is easy to accomplish. If, however, you are using a mug, find a saucer to set atop the mug while your tea steeps. If you are using a mason jar, screw the lid on loosely, so it is not vacuum tight when you try to open it in a few minutes. You are resourceful, if your steep-ware is lidless, you will think of a solution.

6. Allow to steep for 10 minutes. The long steep time infuses the medicinal properties into the water. You can steep the tea for less time if you prefer a mild tasting tea; however, know that it will have little medical properties. You can allow the tea to steep longer, for a stronger tea, too. Experiment and note your preferences regarding flavor, texture (some herbs have a smooth feel, a syrupy texture after prolonged steep - try soaking a broken cinnamon stick in a glass mason jar full of water overnight, and you will see what I mean), and effects on body, mood, and energy, T. Find what you like.

7. Strain and Enjoy!
Some steep-ware make preparing the tea a breeze. A French press, for example, you push down the plunger and pour, voila - strained tea. Others types of steep-ware require the use of a tea strainer (or any strainer, really). You pour the tea through the strainer into the cup to remove bits of leave, or other plant material. Some teapots have a strainer built-in on the inside where the spigot connects to the body of the teapot, others do not, so take a look before you fill the teapot.

Making tea can be a ritual. The very act of preparing the

material, awaiting the boil, handling the steep-ware, and awaiting the infusion can be intention, can be part of finding and experiencing tranquility. The process or preparing the materials and making the tea allows you to slow down and be fully present for a moment. That is a gift. Then when you hold the warm cup in your hand, breath in the aroma, that is another moment building the tranquility. Then the tea itself. Ah. What a wonderful act. A cup of tea.

You can blend catnip with many other herbs to create delicious tea blends. The options are many, and open to your taste and creativity. Make a soothing blend of catnip, chamomile, and passionflower to support relaxation and restful sleep. Combine catnip, fennel, dandelion leaf (or root) for a digestive support tonic.

Share a pot of catnip tea, and expand the effect to community. A simple cup of tea addresses many aspects of wellness. The herb nourishes the body and supports body system function, the ritual of making tea attends spirituality, sharing tea forges connections with others. A pot of tea is an excellent instance of the multi-faceted nature of wellness, and the power of healing inherent in forming personal relationships with plants.

Catnip can be made into a delightful cat treat
Pick of a leaf or stem and give directly to cat
Crush leaf or stem gently to release aromatic constituents
Crumble dried plant material between fingers
Spread on fabric, cardboard scratchpad, toy, or even the floor

While many cats eat the leaves of fresh catnip plant, it is not ingestion that inspires the euphoric reaction. The scent of catnip react with the cats brain. So rubbing or crushing the leaves is enough to inspire a kitty reaction. Know that not all cats are susceptible to the scent of catnip, so watch your cat's reaction to determine its affinity for the plant. Even if they are not euphoric, catnip helps to quell animal anxiety, rub some of the crushed plant on dog or cat alike to help support state-of-mind if the animal seems anxious or stressed.

Pair ginger and catnip to address nausea or queasiness. A recipe that for people or animals.[10]

For example, if you have a child that gets carsick or quest during road-trips, like my niece, then prepare before departure. Make some ginger-catnip tea or pastilles and pack them for refreshment. The beverage blend may be drunk while it is warm or when it is cool. For children over 2 years old, add some honey to sweeten the drink, or, as Mary Poppins sings, "a spoonful of sugar helps the medicine go down, the medicine go down, in the most delightful way." A glass with a straw for sipping is an excellent approach.

Catnip-Ginger blend tea version:
1. Step one Make a decoction of ginger root
Sliced 1 inch of fresh ginger root
Place in pot of 12 oz water
Heat to simmer

---

[10]Wulff-Tilford, Mary, and Gregory Tilford. <u>All YOu Ever Wanted to Know About Herbs for Pets</u>. Bowtie Press, 1999.

Simmer 30 minutes with lid on so water does not evaporate (or start with 18-20 oz water if not have tight fitting lid, still cover pot so constituents remain in water rather than evaporate with steam)

Turn off heat

2. *Step two Make catnip infusion*

Add to ginger infused water 1 heaping tsp catnip

Cover and let sit 10 minutes

Strain and serve

For animals - follow the same procedure as above, though instead of water use bone broth base. Animals are more likely to drink herbs steeped in bone broth. The bone broth makes it much more appealing. You could make a bone broth, ginger, catnip infusion for people, especially if their queasiness is associated with prolonged illness, or chemotherapy effect, because bone broth is nutritious and helps provide healing support.

Catnip-Ginger blend pastille version:

Same idea as tea, only relying on a small, solid pellet-like item to be eaten. Sometimes the pellet will work better for dogs or cats who don't do well in transit.

Many people like these little treats too. You make it into a 'pellet' form, think Pez-like, or a pastille (Altoid for example).

Instructions:

Use powdered form of ginger to make pellet form

Pulverize catnip with mortar and pestle (or coffee grinder)until it is the texture of flour or sugar

Combine catnip powder with the powdered ginger root in a 1 to

1 ratio (1 TBS catnip powder, 1 TBS ginger, for example)
Add drop of honey and roll three ingredients into a little pellet
Eat (or give to pet)

Cautions/Considerations: Do not ingest the seeds! Be sure to harvest plant before seeds begin to form. If you are at all concerned about your timing, then err on the side of harvest before plant is in flower. The leaves and stems provide the constituents even if no flowers are in the blend.

Avoid high doses when pregnant or on pregnant animals. A cup of tea is fine, just not medicinal doses throughout the day.

Notes, comments, questions, drawings... a space for you.

German Chamomile
Matricaria recutita

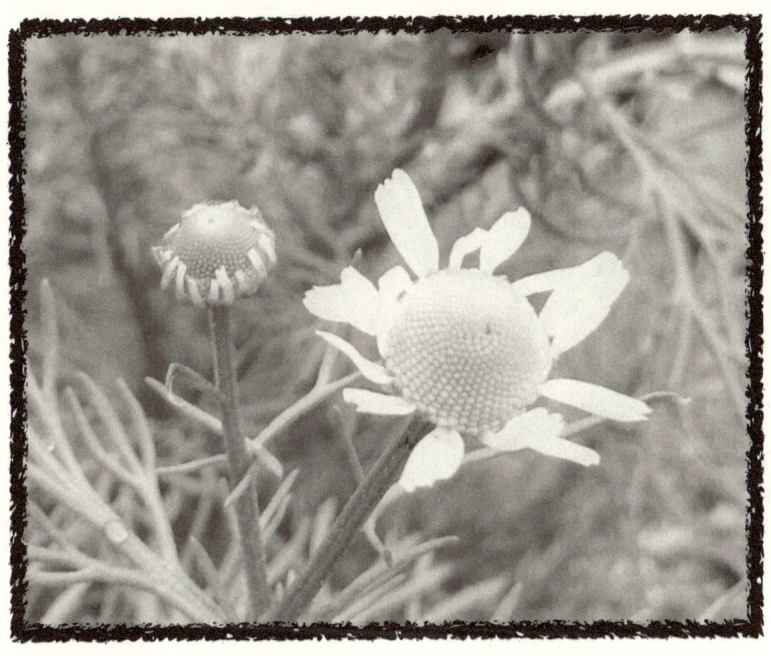

Ah, darling chamomile. Allow me to spend a few paragraphs discussing this popular, powerful plant. As the name German chamomile (Matricaria recutita) implies, it is native to Europe. Now naturalized throughout much of the world as a welcome weed. It is not considered invasive or a threat to native ecosystems. Chamomile grows in disturbed areas such as roadsides, sidewalks, empty lots. The scent is distinctive, so if you are walking along an area populated with stray chamomile, you may be rewarded with its lovely aroma. Manzanilla means little apple, and is chosen as the name for chamomile in Spanish to refer to the small flowers and apple-like scent. In addition to the lovely aroma, the small yellow flowers are cheerful and chummy.

Very few people are unfamiliar with chamomile. Ask most folks and they will share a story of chamomile tea, most likely picturing youth, family, or home. I know that there was always a box of chamomile tea in the tea cupboard amongst the orange pekoe and Lipton black tea. Many different cultures across the globe note a long standing affinity for the unassuming plant. Even a cursory search about the plant confirms that societies from ancient to contemporary value chamomile, or, as my husband fondly refers to it, manzanilla.

Chamomile, renowned a gentle and soothing, serves as an excellent tea for children, to calm or soothe when over-tired or over-stimulated. A study of chamomiles effects to soothe infants with cholic showed a 57% success rate. [11] Brew some chamomile tea, strain it well, allow it to cool, and then put in a bottle for an infant or cup for toddlers and young children.

Chamomile is mild enough for adults as well as children to drink daily to promote quality sleep. You can even add crumbled dried chamomile flowers onto pet foods to soothe agitated dogs or cats (or horses.) The soothing gentle plant is a sunny in disposition as it yellow-centered flower.

The beneficial constituents are packed into those cheerful blooms. (More about harvesting and using chamomile blooms later in the monograph.) The Chamomile Monograph on the

---

[11] Singh, Ompal, et al. "Chamomile (Matricaria Chamomilla L.): An Overview." *Pharmacognosy Reviews*, Medknow Publications Pvt Ltd, Jan. 2011, www.ncbi.nlm.nih.gov/pmc/articles/PMC3210003/.

Herbal Academy Herbarium site lists constituents of chamomile as, "coumarins, flavonoids, glycosides, sesquiterpenes, tannins, quercetin, volatile oils." [12] Each constituent interacts with the human body uniquely, and in combination, synergystically. In other words, the unique constituents influence the impact of one another when they occur together in the whole plant. Some of the wats chamomile supports human systems function include: easing tension and anxiety, stimulating digestive function, reduce abdominal pain or discomfort, reduce inflammation, and even, used topically, clean and support wound healing.

Appreciated the world over, chamomile asserts its gentle presence in many cultures. "Herbs for Health", by Stephen Foster reports that a Slovakian chamomile specialist, Ivan Salamon, says, "Chamomile is the most favored and most used medicinal plant in Slovakia. Our folk saying that an individual should always bow when facing a chamomile plant. This respect results from hundreds of years experience with [chamomile]."[13] "Spanish speakers often refer to [chamomile] as Manzanilla, and it is probably the most popular herb among Latin Americans, who use it to reduce stress and anxiety and relieve minor GI complaints," explains Dr. Sierpina nor Dr. Loera, two physicians collaborating on a book to "help educate non-Hispanic health

12 "The Herbarium." *The Herbarium,* Herbal Academy, herbarium.theherbalacademy.com/monographs/#/monograph/1.

13Foster, Stephen. *Herbs for Your Health: A Handy Guide for Knowing and Using 50 Common Herbs.* Interweave Press, 1996 care professionals about Hispanic herbal practices.[14]

In addition to the many wonderful herbal concoctions and wellness supporting benefits of chamomile, the plant is a welcome addition to the garden with its lacy leaves and abundant bright flowers, chamomile offer more than its beauty and grace. The medicinal properties of chamomile include its tendency to soothe the nerves, ease digestion, support restful sleep, promote wound healing, calm inflammation, and ease stress. Grow and befriend this dynamic little plant.

Grow, tend, and garden befriend

Chamomile grows well with little effort on the part of the gardener, offers cheery blooms and lovely foliage, enhances the growth of other plants, and offers abundant support to wellness, all excellent reasons to add chamomile to your yarden.

Growing Conditions

Chamomile grows as an annual in U.S. plant hardiness zones 2 - 8, meaning it lives only a single season. However, chamomile does grow and flower abundantly during the growing season. As a bonus, in my opinion, chamomile often will reseed itself, and grow the following year. I experienced the reseed benefit in both a garden plot and in containers. During summer as I pass the chamomile patch in my garden, I am amazed by how

---

[14] Writer, Staff. â€œA Guide to Hispanic Healing Herbs.â€Â *Holistic Primary Care*, 1 Dec. 2009, www.holisticprimarycare.net/topics/topics-o-z/traditions/210-a-guide-to-hispanic-healing-herbs.html.

quickly the chamomile plant grows and how abundantly it blooms.

I stop and stoop to brush the lacy leaves and take in that delightful scent of the bloom.

Chamomile is a member of the Aster (Asteraceae) family, and shares characteristics with plants like the sunflower and dandelion. The inflorescence is especially noteworthy. What we think of as the chamomile flower, is really a cluster of many flowers arranged in such a way that they appear to be a single larger flower. In fact, chamomile has 2 distinct types of flowers in the inflorescence: ray flowers and disc flowers. While the entire inflorescence is small, you can get a good look by using a magnifying lens or field glass. If you do look closely, and it is easier to tell on a larger flower of the aster family, like the sunflower, you will be able to distinguish the parts. Ray flowers are the parts that look like the traditional concept of a flower petal. The white petals of the chamomile are ray flowers. The yellow conical center comprise the disc flowers. Each flower may make seed, so the chamomile inflorescence produces many seeds. Think about how many sunflower seeds are in a sunflower head, and you may imagine what I mean.

Not a 'fussy' plant, chamomile thrives in many gardens. Chamomile grows well in many soil types, and especially thrives in light sandy soil.[15] Rich soil produces more lush foliage, but doe not necessarily result in more flower blooms. Chamomile flowers are both more prolific and more potent

---

[15]*Matricaria Recutita - Plant Finder*, www.missouribotanicalgarden.org/PlantFinder/PlantFinderDetails.aspx?taxonid=277347.

when grown in less-rich soil. In other words, chamomile is well-suited to less than ideal nutrient content in soil.

While growing well in a wide range of situations, chamomile will tend to get leggy in very hot weather.

Preferences:

Dry, light, well-drained soil

Full sun

Tolerates wide range of pH[16]

Shallow roots, so water during dry stretches

Plant details

1 to 2 feet in height

Bushy, yet spreading growth (wider than tall, often)

Companion Planting Affiliations: Chamomile enhances the growth of cucumbers, onions, and most other herbs, so plant it amongst beds with other herbs. It does spread, so allot it some space, or keep and eye on it.

Rosemary Gladstar, a 'grandmother' to the world of modern herbalism in America, shares in her book, Medicinal Herbs: A Beginners Guide, that chamomile is recognized by gardeners as an excellent companion plant that is known to keep neighboring plants, "healthy and disease free."[17]

I sprout seeds of various plants in late winter. Seed trays are vulnerable to a fungal infection called 'damping off'. When I saw a few young plants show symptoms, I removed them from

[16] Singh, Ompal, et al. â€œChamomile (Matricaria Chamomilla L.): An Overview.â€Â *Pharmacognosy Reviews*, Medknow Publications Pvt Ltd, Jan. 2011, www.ncbi.nlm.nih.gov/pmc/articles/PMC3210003/.

[17]Gladstar, Rosemary. *Medicinal Herbs: A Beginner's Guide.* Storey Publishing, 2012

the sprout room and sprayed all the remaining seed trays with a chamomile tea solution. Chamomile is anti-fungal, and serves as an excellent organic strategy to combat damping off. I am happy to report the treatment was a success, and easy apply.

Care notes: Chamomile grows well both in the ground and in containers. So, if your space is limited, you can still grow and befriend a chamomile plant or three. Try planting seeds or transplanting a chamomile start in a flowerpot, hanging basket, or window-box.

Ways the plants support wellness

I often turn to the gentle balm of chamomile when I am tired but can't sleep, anxious and yearn for calm, feel a rumbly in my tummy, after a meal to ease digestion, and so many other moments where I long for support. Many body systems benefit from the soothing strains of chamomile, which is mild enough to drink daily as a tonic, yet useful in acute situations as well. I think the more you learn about chamomile, the more you will both respect and admire it. I really liked chamomile to begin with, and the more time I spend with the plant, interact with it in herbal concoctions, hear others discuss its attributes, and research it, the deeper my appreciation and respect for this well known plant becomes.

Actions: carminative, sedative, bitter, antidepressant, hypnotic, cholagogue, anti-microbial

Energetics: neutral to cooling, moistening[18]

Consituents: "dried chamomile, the flowers in particular, contain a large amount of hydrophilic constituents (sugars, flavonoids, mucilages, phenyl carbonic acids, amino acids, choline, salts)"[19]

Chamomile as a nervine: Juliet Blankespoor explains, in her course "Herbal Immersion" that chamomile is a mild hypnotic. She explains, "Hypnotic herbs help induce or sustain deep sleep. They can be taken right before bedtime to encourage sleepiness or in the middle of the night to help you go back to sleep."[20] Chamomile's mildness makes it safe to use with children and elders.

Chamomile is also considered an anxiolytic, which means it reduces anxiety. Such an effect on the nervous system is best achieved by taking the herb tonically, or as a daily dose over time.

Chamomile support the nervous system as a gentle analgesic, which means it relieves pain.

As you can see, chamomile is an excellent friend to the nervous system, soothing, calming, and easing the cells or the function of the nervous system.

---

[18]Johnson, Jackie. "Get to Know the Versatile Chamomile Plant - Herbal Academy Blog." *Herbal Academy*, 25 Jan. 2018, theherbalacademy.com/get-to-know-the-versatile-chamomile-plant/.

[19] Singh, Ompal, et al. â€œChamomile (Matricaria Chamomilla L.): An Overview.â€Â *Pharmacognosy Reviews*, Medknow Publications Pvt Ltd, Jan. 2011, www.ncbi.nlm.nih.gov/pmc/articles/PMC3210003/.

[20]Blanekespoor, Juliet. "Herbal Immersion Program." *Chestnut School of Herbal Medicine*, Herbal Immersion Program,chestnutherbs.com/lesson/introduction-to-nervines-hypnotics-anxiolytics-antidepressants-and-analgesics/.

Parts Used: Flowers

When to Harvest: when flower is in full bloom

When the chamomile flowers in my garden were fully open and fragrant the moment for me to make my first chamomile harvest arrived. I read many suggestions instructing to 'use fingers to gently rake' the open blooms of the flowers into a basket. Yeah, right. I tried. I failed; I found that the suggestion to gently rake with fingers is not as easy to do as it sounds. I ended up using sharp scissors to snip close to the flower head; very close, because only the flower is the medicinal part. A little bit of stem won't hurt you, but it is easier to take the time to harvest well before drying rather than trying to separate stems out afterward, and preferable to having chamomile blooms diluted by the presence of dried stem.

Flowers of varying stages of development, bud, just opening, mature, transitioning to seed, will all be on the plant at the same time, so be observant while harvesting. The medicinal constituent content is most concentrated in the flower at peak bloom. Do not pick flowers that have transitioned to seed. Look for the white petals and bright yellow conical center.

Use the harvested chamomile flowers fresh or dried. You can dry the flower by spreading thinly on mesh trays or baskets left to sit in a dark place with regular adequate air circulation. A shed, attic, or other dry, dark space with air circulation is ideal. If the climate or environment is damp or without air flow, I suggest using a food dehydrator, if you have one. The dehydrator will drastically speed the drying process, thus lower the risk of mold developing before the flower heads dry. If you do not have, nor want to purchase a food dehydrator, another option for drying herbs is to use your car. Arranging paper bags containing herbs in my car windowsill is my current favorite drying method. Place the chamomile flowers in a paper bag, take care that the flowers aren't stacked thickly atop each other. Remember - air flow is important to the drying process. Airflow reduces to possibility for mold to grow on the plant material. Roll the bag closed, like a lunch bag. Then place the closed paper bag on the dashboard of your car. Allow it to sit a few hours or a day or two, and presto, dried chamomile flowers. A wonderful benefit of this particular drying method is your car smelling of herbs. Check the bags of herbs occasionally to determine when the plant material is sufficiently dry. Generally, especially with leaf parts, when the plant material crumbles easily in your hand and makes a sort of crunch or crinkle sound, then it is sufficiently dried. Put them immediately into an airtight container. Herbs are stored in airtight containers to prevent them from absorbing moisture and spoiling. All the effort of growing and tending the plant, harvesting and drying the material warrants care in storage. In addition to keeping them dry, the longevity of the herb is protected if they are stored out of light and away from heat. Heat and light causes the constituent concentration within the herb to deteriorate. Stored well, herbs may last a year, or a bit more and retain viable constituents.

The chamomile growing in my garden plot blooms so

abundantly that I harvest blooms every few days. I leave some blooms on the plant for pollinators, and to set seed. The others I dry for later herbal preparations.

How to Prepare

Chamomile flowers make an excellent tea.

The Herbal Academy Blog discusses the virtues of chamomile tea. "If you're using chamomile for stress, a mild tea should suffice. A stronger version would be used for sleep. If you steep chamomile too long, however, the tea may become bitter, so taste it first before drinking it."[21] What this quote references is the time steeping determines the concentration of the medicinal constituents in the resulting tisane (tea). If you are drinking the chamomile infusion on a regular basis throughout the day, or daily, then a milder infusion will serve you. If, however, you want a stronger dose to alleviate acute anxiety or stress before going to sleep, then a longer infusion will have a greater impact on the nervous system. Be aware, the flavor will be different too. Long infusions of chamomile extract more of the bitter properties, and result in a more bitter infusion. If you have over-steeped tea, black or green, then you are familiar with how the resulting flavor takes on a noticeably bitter flavor. Contrary to what common attitude asserts, bitter is neither undesirable nor unpalatable. Bitter is an important flavor for our bodies, conveying both information and catalyzing action. Your ability

---

[21] Johnson, Jackie. â€œGet to Know the Versatile Chamomile Plant - Herbal Academy Blog.â€Â *Herbal Academy*, 25 Jan. 2018, theherbalacademy.com/get-to-know-the-versatile-chamomile-plant/.

to effectively digest food and absorb nutrients is connected to bitters. Chamomile is considered a mild bitter. The longer chamomiles steeped the more the bitter notes extract. Keep notes of your tea steeping and flavor profiles, recognizing your flavor preferences, and the action the tea has on your body. By noting details and nuances, you can learn much about how to prepare tea particularly suited to you.

In addition to time steeped, another factor that influences strength of resulting brew is the amount of herb you use in making the infusion. Experiment with the variables, though keeping records is key to drawing conclusions.

I personally enjoy a strong infusion of chamomile. Often, I use chamomile blooms in a blend, so the flavor is combined with other herbs for a synergistic whole. Blending herbs tends to enhance the impact on the body. The various herbs in the blend compliment of counter-balance each other.

Sometimes I make a mild chamomile tea, and sip it hot; other times I make a strong infusion, and drink that. Still other times I make an especially potent infusion, allowing the chamomile to steep until it is nearly cool, then pour it over ice and enjoy. I drink chamomile in one form or another most days.

Tea making:
For a very descriptive discussion on making herbal tea see either the catnip monograph, or herbal blends section of this book.

1. Boil water (or heat to just before boiling point)
The blog post mentioned above by the Herbal Academy advises not to boil the water, or "the aromatics can be destroyed."

2. Place 2 tsp of fresh chamomile flowers or 1 tsp of dried chamomile flowers per 8 oz water into teapot, press, thermos, or mason jar.

3. Pour boiling water over blooms

4. Cover (this is very important, for if uncovered the constituents will rise with the steam, and you will have a less flavorful, less potent cup of chamomile tea)

5. Allow to steep for 10 minutes
        or your preferred steeping time

6. Strain and Enjoy!

You can blend chamomile with many other herbs to create delicious tea blends. Try chamomile and ginger root, chamomile and lemon balm, chamomile, peppermint, ginger. The options are many, and open to your taste and creativity.

Chamomile can be made into tasty treats!

Katja Swift of Commonwealth Center of Holistic Herbalism, in Boston, Massachusetts shares her recipe for Ginger Chamomile Cookies; you can find the full post on the Commonwealth Herbs Blog.

Recipe:

    1. Preheat oven to 350 degrees Fahrenheit

    2. Mix with a fork into a thick, doughy batter:

        1 cup almond meal

        1 cup shredded coconut

        ~2/3 cup coconut oil

        1/4 cup honey

        1 egg

        1 tsp cinnamon

        Salt

    3. Add to above batter:

        2/3 cup chopped candied ginger.

        2 to 3 tablespoons dried chamomile

Ginger preparation notes:

Katja recommends, "I like to candy my own ginger – I get local fresh young ginger rhizomes and chop them, then put them in a mason jar and cover them with honey. in a month or two, candied ginger! (store in the fridge)"

Chamomile notes:

Pour dried chamomile into a strainer and sift to get the tiny bits. Replace the chamomile that did not fall through the sifter to the chamomile jar.

1. Mix batter again.
2. Spoon onto baking tray, or roll into a ball and flatten
3. Bake 350 for 20-30 minutes.

Katja concludes with "They're delicious, low-carb, gluten and dairy free, and downright good for you!"[22]

Chamomile as a anti-fungal garden spray

As I noted earlier in the monograph, I used chamomile infusion as a spray to combat damping-off. Below is a summary of the process.

1. Steep an especially potent chamomile infusion
In a tempered glass jar, like a Mason jar, I steeped 1 cup of chamomile flowers in 2 quarts of water. I placed a lid on the jar and let it sit overnight.
By next morning, the water temperature is cooled and the infusion is strong.

2. Strain infusion well
Next I strained the liquid carefully through a fine mesh strainer lined with fine cheese cloth.

---

[22]Swift, Katja."Ginger Chamomile Cookies." *Commonwealth Herbs Blog*. Commonwealth Center of Holistic Herbalism. December 9, 2016. https://commonwealthherbs.com/ginger-chamomile-cookies/

Since I will apply it as a spray, I don't want any plant material clogging the sprayer.

3. Apply on plant starts and soil tray
I pour the well-strained liquid into a pump sprayer, foliar applicator. I then add another quart of water to the pump sprayer. I mist all the flats with the chamomile infusion. I repeated the application in the evening, if I had any chamomile infusion remaining in the bottle.

Use all the liquid in 24 hours, or it will begin to spoil.

Cautions/Considerations

Chamomile is a very safe plant; however, some people are allergic to chamomile. If you get itchy eyes or ears, a runny nose, a scratchy-throat, or other allergy signs, discontinue use of chamomile.
Avoid using chamomile as or in a blend as an eyewash. The pollen in the flowers may cause an allergic reaction if the eye is bathed in a chamomile based eyewash.[23]

[23] Singh, Ompal, et al. â€œChamomile (Matricaria Chamomilla L.): An Overview.â€Â *Pharmacognosy Reviews*, Medknow Publications Pvt Ltd, Jan. 2011, www.ncbi.nlm.nih.gov/pmc/articles/PMC3210003/.

Notes, comments, questions, drawings... a space for you.

Lavender
Lavendula angustifolia
'English lavender'

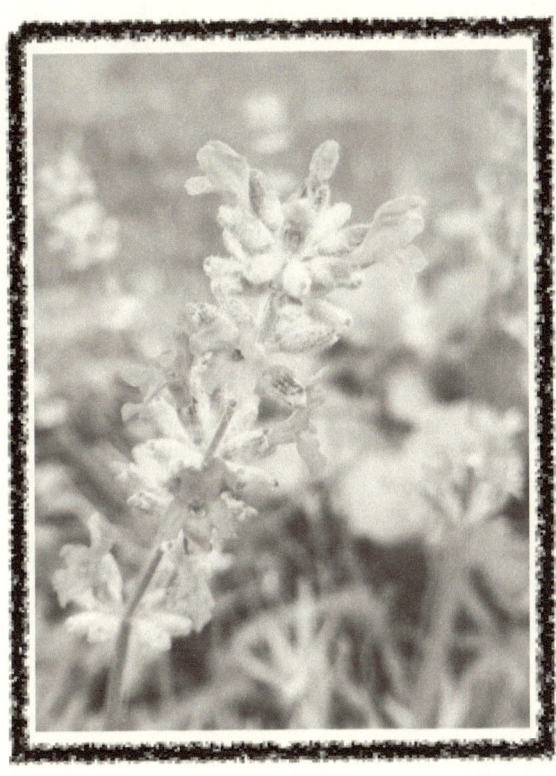

Tiny purple flowers arranged on a slender sprig, narrow blue-green leaves reminiscent of an evergreen, and a delicate sweet scent are some of lavender's attributes. Brush the soft leaves with your hand to release a recognizable scent that carries with it calmness for spirit and a lift to the mood. I love lavender. I keep a sachet of lavender leaves under my pillow to support sound sleep. I drop flowers from a single sprig into with my jasmine green tea before it steeps. I watch the small pollinators alight on the blooms. I spend hours appreciating the wonders of this perennial plant. While there are many species of lavender, and even more cultivars, In my yarden I grow Lavandula angustafolia, sometimes referred to as 'English Lavender', though it is not native to England.

Lavender has a long history in herbalism, used for a variety of applications from spiritual to topical in many cultures from Greece, Egypt, and ancient Rome to contemporary Germany, England and America.

Lavender is associated with cleanliness, even in name, linked in origin to the Latin word, *lavare*, meaning to wash. Historically associated with lavender water, a means of sweetening the scent of linens or person.

Lavender also has a history of culinary use, from flavored breads to butters, and desserts. <u>The Pleasures of Tea: Recipes and Rituals</u> includes a recipe for both lavender tea and lavender sorbet.[24]

I love lavender, the plant, the flower, the scent. I stop by my lavender bushes and rub the leaves to release the scent. The aromatic scent brings me joy, what a generous offering. I like watching the tiny pollinators fly about the lavender flower stalks. The slender, silvery leaves are so different from everything else growing around it.

Lavender is a friend to the nervous system. Lavender offers much to the home - antimicrobial properties that make it useful in cleaning, aroma that is soothing and calming, support for

---

24 Waller, Kim. The Pleasures of Tea: Recipes and Rituals. Hearst Books, 1999.

liver and digestive systems, delightful flavor for recipes… the contexts suitable to the strains of lavender are many indeed. No wonder so many cultures associate with it, no wonder it has traveled so far from its home. I dream of standing in a field full of lavender someday. In bloom or not, it will be glorious.

Grow, tend, and garden befriend

Growing Conditions

Originating from a Mediterranean clime, lavender thrives when situated in full sun with well-draining soil. Lavender will bloom in early to mid-summer, attracting butterflies, small bees, and other pollinators to its blooms. Even when finished flowering, the soft-hued blue-green leaves still provide a lovely edition to garden bed or border.

A fan of an arid climate, lavender struggles with wet, stagnant conditions. Juliet Blankespoor, of Chestnut School of Herbal Medicine, notes on her blog Castanea, "Try mulching with sand, light-colored gravel or oyster shells if you live near the sea. High humidity and cold wet winters can be problematic." Juliet adds, "If your native soil doesn't drain well, try adding gravel or rocks to the soil."

Lavender is a perennial, dying back and regrowing from roots in cold climates, and becoming shrubby in warm climates with mild winters. Lavender is a member of the mint family, yet is not an overly-assertive grower. Lavender tends to stay well contained where planted rather than tenaciously taking over garden beds.

Preferences

Full sun

Tolerates drought (once established)

Prefers well drained soil

Tolerates rocky soil[25]

Plant details *vary by cultivar

    Flowers small purple blooms on mid-summer

    Repeat blooms if trim flower stalks

    Height to 2 ft in cool climates where die back annually

        (mine are smaller, not quite a foot, and this

          is their 3rd year)

    To 3 foot in warm climates where gets shrubby

    Width 1 foot (mine have spread wider than tall)

Companion Planting Affiliations

Lavender's "scent attracts pollinators [and] repels several types of beetles and flies, as well as mice and rabbits."[26] The same article goes on to say that lavender makes "an excellent companion to broccoli, cabbage, kale, and cauliflower because it doesn't compete with them for nutrients."

Lavender provides as an excellent border plant for herb and vegetable beds due to its growth habit, and its companion planting benefits.

[25]"Lavandula Angustifolia (English Lavender)." *Gardenia.net*, www.gardenia.net/plant-variety/lavandula-angustifolia-english-lavender.

[26]Wilson, Rickie. "Companion Planting with Herbs." *Herb Quarterly*, 2018, pp. 48–52.

Care notes: Once established, lavender requires little water thus will tolerate dry conditions or an inattentive gardener. However, lavender is sensitive to excess, so do not plant in heavy clay soils (without amendments) or locations that are wet or slow to drain. If you have that kind of spot in your yarden, chose an herb better suited to the conditions. Prairie Nursery, which specializes in native plants, recommends boneset (*Eupatorium perfoliatum*), or *Monarda fistulosa*, among others, as excellent options of plants suited to succeed in moist conditions.[27] Choosing the right site for each plant increases the likelihood the plant will thrive.

Lavender flourishes in the sun, so place it where it will get many hours of sunlight. Lavender's love of light and excellent drainage, makes it a fine candidate for a sunny hillside.

If your conditions for lavender are less than ideal, augment heavy soils by adding sand, and Taylor's Guide to Herbs advices, "plant 'high' by positioning the crown above the surrounding grade so water will run away from the plant.[28]

The Sunset National Garden Book states that lavender requires little to no fertilizer. Lavender is a self-sufficient plant. I still suggest feeding the soil, use mulch, add compost, respect the soil microbiome.

---

[27] "Plant Finder." *Prairie Nursery*, www.prairienursery.com/store/native-plants/bergamot-monarda-fistulosa#.XhHkP-t7mi4.

[28]Buchanan, Rita. *Taylor's Guide to Herbs*. Houghton Mifflin, 1995.

Ways the plants support wellness

Lavender is a nervine, an herb that supports healthy functions of nerves and the nervous system. Juliet Blankespoor, of Chestnut School of Herbal Medicine, explains, "Lavender is a gentle sedative and can help with anxiety, stress and insomnia. It is often used in formula for the herbal treatment of depression as it has more immediate effects as compared to many of the slower-acting tonic antidepressants and adaptogens."[29] Lavender finds favor and fame in the world of aromatherapy. The scent of lavender lifts the mood, elevates emotion, and supports soothing grief. Lavender scent supports restful sleep; a sachet of lavender leaf and flower, sometimes combined with other herbs, sometimes solo, kept by your pillow helps you find your way to and remain in the land of nod.

As wonderful as I find the scent of lavender, it is made even more positive by the fact that many insects are repelled by the scent. Yippee! WIth the help of lavender, mosquitoes and ticks are kept at bay. I make insect repelling jewelry, yes I said jewelry. I use essential oils, including lavender with lemon eucalyptus, or peppermint, or other insect repellent scents. I dab a drop of each oil on a leather anklet and a leather bracelet. "Recharging" the jewelry as the scent fades by reapplying a drop of each essential oil.

Additionally to supporting nervous system, lavender supports

---

[29]Blankespoor, Juliet. "Lavender's Medicinal and Aromatherapy Uses." *Chestnut School of Herbal Medicine*, 1 May 2018, chestnutherbs.com/lavenders-medicinal-and-aromatherapy-uses-and-lavender-truffles/.

digestive function through its slightly bitter flavor that stimulates bile and its carminative effect, helping to prevent and relates gas build-up in the intestines. Lavender is also a friend to the immune system. The anti-fungal and anti-microbial actions support the work of the immune system in its ever-vigilant approach to fending off infection.

So much goodness in such a lovely smelling and aesthetically pleasing plant.

Actions: antidepressant, anti-fungal, anti-microbial, antispasmodic, bitter, carminative, cholagogue, diuretic, hypnotic, nervine, sedative,

Energetics: drying, cooling

As a nervine: When I see lavender, plant and bloom, I immediately smile. I associate the plant with calm joy and peace of mind. I do not think I am alone in this association. The HerbRally lavender monograph states, "In ritual use, lavender often represents love, protection and purification."[30]

These associations speak to the interaction lavender has with the human nervous system. The HerbRally lavender monograph goes on to explain, "[Lavender] is incredibly relaxing to the nervous system. Just the aroma itself can help reduce stress and anxiety in most people."

Pairing lavender with other nervine herbs creates effective results. For example, lavender partners perfectly with chamomile in a calming tea or for an herbal bath.

---

[30]Hazard, Sara. "Lavender Monograph." *HerbRally*, www.herbrally.com/monographs/lavender.

Parts Used: flowers and leaves[31]

When to Harvest : Harvest while plant is in bloom

Harvest the flower stalk just as the flowers are about to open, preferably mid to late morning, after the dew has evaporated, but before the heat of the day stresses the plant and lessens the concentration of constituents present in the flower stalk.

How to Prepare

Though lavender is most often thought of because of its delightful scent, the plant possessed many other facets to its herbal profile. Lavender boasts many topical uses, and is also an ally to internal body systems. So, find a use suited to the situation, and get to know the many wonders of lavender.

As a recipe

Add fresh lavender flowers to baked goods, or to flavor ice cream suggests <u>Taylor's Guide to Herbs</u>. Other lavender recipe options are noted in <u>Rodale's Illustrated Encyclopedia of Herbs,</u> which suggests "when making apple jelly or raspberry jam, add a sprig of lavender to each jar."[32]

As a tea [enhancement or in blend]

While, I don't drink a tea of lone lavender, I do love to add lavender to a blend. The flavor of lavender is strong; a little

---

[31]Gladstar, Rosemary. *Herbs for Stress & Anxiety: How to Make and Use Herbal Remedies to Strengthen the Nervous System.* Storey Publishing, 2014.

[32]Kowalchik, Claire, and William H. Hylton. *Rodale's Illustrated Encyclopedia of Herbs: Editors.* Rodale Press, 1987.

lavender provides a lot of flavor. Too much lavender overpowers a tea blend and becomes unpalatable.

Juliet Blankespoor, of Chestnut School of Herbal Medicine, shares the following about lavender, as a tea:

> "Preparation & Dosage:1-2 teaspoons (approximately .8 to 1.6 grams) of the flower or herb with flower per 8 ounces of water as an infusion, drink up to three times a day.
> I combine lavender with lemon balm (Melissa officinalis) and lemon verbena (Aloysia citrodora) in tea to help lift the spirits. Lavender is also used to alleviate grief; it is often paired with the flowers of hawthorn (Crataegus spp.), rose (Rosa spp.), and mimosa (Albizia julibrissin).
> Lavender is a traditional remedy for headaches; both internally as a tea and externally as an essential oil, rubbed into the temples.
> Notes: The flavor of lavender tea is stronger than one might expect: slightly bitter, mildly astringent and very aromatic. A little goes a long way"[33]

To make an herbal tea, infuse the herb in boiling water, which will extract many of the beneficial constituents. Begin

---

[33]Blankespoor, Juliet. "Lavender's Medicinal and Aromatherapy Uses." *Chestnut School of Herbal Medicine*, 1 May 2018, chestnutherbs.com/lavenders-medicinal-and-aromatherapy-uses-and-lavender-truffles/.

by boiling (or near boiling, depending on your preference) water. As you await the water to heat, place 2 tsp of the dried herb blend you combined per 8 oz water into teapot, press, thermos, or mason jar. When the water is heated to the desired temperature, pour the water over the herbs in the selected steep-ware container. Place a cover on the steep-ware container immediately to ensure the desired herbal constituents infuse into the water rather than evaporating with the steam. Allow the teapot (or press, or mason jar) of water and herbs to steep for 10 minutes then strain and enjoy the delightful brew.

For a tasty morning tea treat, I add a 1/2 teaspoon of dried lavender blooms to the teapot for a second steeping of my jasmine tea. I start my day by brewing a small pot of loose leaf jasmine tea. Then, I make a second pot using the same jasmine green tea leaves, still in the teapot, and add a 1/2 teaspoon of dried lavender blooms, or in summer, a single sprig of fresh lavender. The resulting tea has a subtle jasmine flavor with notes of lavender. If you like earl grey tea, I think you may like jasmine second steep with lavender.
I also throw it into many other herbal blends I make. I currently find lavender to be a very good friend indeed. Here are a few blend ideas to try: chamomile, tulsi, and lavender; rose petal and lavender; catnip, lemon balm, chamomile, and lavender; green tea and lavender; or earl grey and lavender. You may even find a pre-made blend in the regular grocery store these days. Lavender, you have made it main-stream.

Experiment, and boldly create your own herbal blends.

As a wound cleaner

If the wound is minor, and you are able to tend it at home, you can use lavender infused water as a wash. Lavender is antiseptic[34], and will help to kill pathogens that might cause infection. Additionally, lavender decreases inflammation and speeds healing[35], a trifecta of attributes.

I am not a medical practitioner. No suggestions in this text constitute medical advice. You are responsible for each and all choices regarding your medical care. This discussion is intended as educational information for you to consider and research further. If you are not sure how to clean a wound, consider taking a first aid class. Obviously, if the wound is serious or severe, seek immediate medical attention.

1. Make an infusion of lavender
2. After steeping for 10 - 15 minutes, you want a good strong infusion when using for a wound wash, strain the herbs from the liquid. Strain well! You do not want any plant material getting into a wound.
3. Soak a clean cotton cloth, or sterile bandage, in the lavender infused water that you have already strained. You do not want to introduce any plant material into a wound

---

[34]McIntyre, Anne. *Herbal Remedies for Everyday Living*. Bounty, 2015.

[35]Groves, Maria Noël. *Body into Balance: an Herbal Guide to Holistic Self-Care*. Storey Publishing, 2016.

4. Clean the wound by either or

    a. by dabbing with the cotton cloth

    b. by rinsing the wound with the lavender water once it has cooled.

As a soak

Add sprigs of fresh lavender to the bath and enjoy a fragrant soak. This is especially lovely to relax before bed, or if you have difficulty falling asleep.

Place a few sprigs (6 or 7) tied with string into the bathtub as you fill it with warm water, the scent of lavender will carry on the warm air, imbuing the room with a peaceful calm. Medicinal properties of the lavender will also be infused in the water. As you soak in the warm bath, you will absorb the effects of lavender through the skin, and by breathing it. The warm water will also relax your muscles, thereby relieving tension. An excellent strategy before bedtime. Add some epsom salts to the water, and enhance the muscle relaxation.

If you only have loose lavender, then you can also use a muslin bag filled with loose lavender. Hang the bag on the spigot so the water flows through it, thus enhancing the extraction of lavender constituents.

As a sachet or sleep pillow

Fill a small muslin or cotton, any breathable cloth, with lavender leaf and bloom, and place under or on your pillow. The scent will help you fall asleep, and will promote deeper sleep. Ah. Sweet dreams. You can blend the lavender with hops, chamomile, or rose to make a wonderful blend that enhances sleep quality.

Cautions/Considerations

If using lavender in essential oil form, then do not ingest. Essential oils are highly concentrated and potent, and are not suited to be taken internally. Do your due diligence when using essential oils; they are a valuable resource for supporting wellness, come with specific safety considerations, and require a high plant content to generate a very small amount of resulting oil. I am not saying do not use essential oils. I have some and use them with consideration. When possible, I opt for the crude herb (plant material that I make directly into teas, tisanes, or tinctures).

Notes, comments, questions, drawings... a space for you.

Lemon Balm
Melissa officinalis

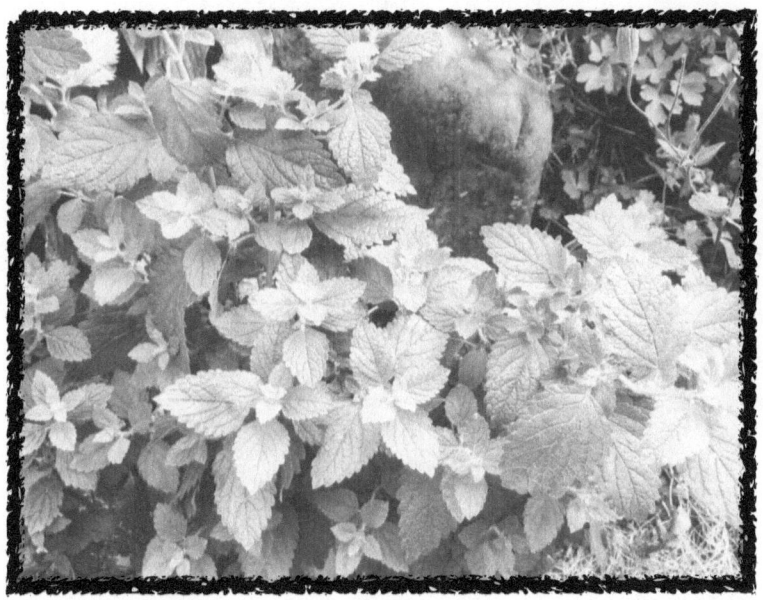

One mid-summer, I moved into our current home and was astounded by the abundance of lemon balm growing on the property. Lush and large lemon balm dominated the river-rock strewn plantings, beds along the house, and even creeping into in the lawn. Lemon balm was confidently popping up virtually everywhere boasting its attributes as an assertive grower, like many mint family plants are. The lemon balm was well-established and comfortably spreading every which where. I harvested a bountiful crop, dried, and stored it. Over the winter I shared the bounty with friends.

Lemon balm has many positive attributes, including a subtle

lemony-flavor and the capacity to sooth to the nervous system. I don't drink much lemon balm because I have a hypo-thyroid condition, and lemon balm can impact the thyroid in a 'slowing' or 'calming' capacity, which is not helpful to me. I do, on occasion, drink tea blends with lemon balm. I find the flavor of lemon balm especially delightful in a spritzer or iced tea.

Lemon balm is easy to grow, so, if a timid or novice gardener, lemon balm eases the way into successful gardening. Put it in a pot or the ground, it does well in either; full-sun, part-shade, also both. Dry conditions, no problem if it is an established plant and in the ground (in a container, drought is another ballyhoo entirely).

Grow, tend, and garden befriend

Growing Conditions: Lemon balm makes a great thick growing bed of plants. Its easygoing nature makes it a good plant for the not-yet-confident gardener. Lemon balm's easy-going nature will tolerate a wide range of conditions, and rewards with a lemony scent, beautiful lush green leaves and delicate tiny blooms. Lemon balm is a confidant perennial to zone 4.

Preferences:

Moist soil

Fun sun to part shade

Neutral pH (7.0)

Plant details:

Height 2 to 3 feet

Width up to 2 feet, spreads abundantly

Tiny white to yellow flowers in July

Companion Planting Affiliations: Bees are fond of lemon balm, thus benefitting the blooming plants growing near lemon balm. My next-door neighbor keeps bee hives, and many a day my lemon balm boast a host of bees hovering about the leaves and blooms. I love watching them bob and dance about.

Care notes: Since lemon balm is an assertive grower, you might want to control it with limits; for example plant it in a raised bed, a bed with edging, or a container. Or Dig it up and share with a friend when it pops up beyond where you prefer it to grow.

Ways the plants support wellness

Energetics: Cold, dry sour, slightly bitter.

Actions: *Nervine*: acts on the nerves. *Sedative*: calming agent. *Mild Antidepressant*: relieves feelings of depression. *Mild Antispasmodic*: reduces voluntary or involuntary muscle spasm. *Carminative*: gently calms the nerves. *Diaphoretic*: Induces perspiration. Lemon balm is a relaxing diaphoretic as opposed to a stimulating diaphoretic. *Antiviral*: destroys or suppresses growth of viruses, generally by supporting the immune system. *Antioxidant*: prevents free radical or oxidative damage.[36]

As you see, lemon balms supports a wide variety of human system function. Part of lemon balm's action results from the aromatic constituents, the volatile oils linalool and citronellol. From the moment you smell the scent of lemon balm, through the ingestion of tea, various effects occur on your nervous system. In an article about aromatics, Urban Moonshine, a women-run organic herbal apothecary focused on quality of product and access to herbal medicine, explains, "may be part of our aromatic herbs' mechanism of action, but in the end, what matters is that a warm cup of aromatic tea first engages your senses, and then supports healthy tone of the smooth muscle in our GI tract and other muscles in our body."[37]

Imagine that, your sense of smell creates a strong link to plants, and plant action begins with scent. Then, your mucous membranes in the gastrointestinal tract take the interaction to the next level when you drink the tea made from lemon balm. A balance of tone is reached in the muscles, a relaxing of spasming balanced with a smooth tightening. Balance.

Parts Used: **Leaves**

When to Harvest:
Harvest ongoing for immediate use. You can make delightful

---

[36] Seitzman, Sara.Seitzman. Lemon Balm Monograph. *HerbRally*, www.herbrally.com/monographs/lemon-balm.

[37] Urban Moonshine, Guido Mase. â€œAromatic Herbs for Stress and Mood.*Urban Moonshine*, 13 Dec. 2018, www.urbanmoonshine.com/blogs/blog/aromatic-herbs-for-stress-and-mood.

tea, iced or hot, from a handful of fresh leaves plucked from the plant.

You can also cut the lemon balm stalks back in early summer for a large crop of leaves to dry. The plant will grow back again, and fuller, providing for another harvest in late summer. Bundle the stems and hang to dry in a dark, warm, dry location with ample air circulation. I made some how-to dry lemon balm youtube videos you can watch.[38]

How to Prepare

There are many ways to use lemon balm to support wellness.

___

As a compress

Use a clean soft cotton cloth soaked in a strong infusion of lemon balm to relieve painful swellings (e.g. gout)

___

As an infused oil

Use dried lemon balm when making an infused oil to lessen the risk the oil will be spoiled. The high water content in fresh herb makes the shelf-life of infused oil shorter, and increases the potential for mold or mildew growth. If you do opt to use fresh leaves, crush or chop them first, and know the shelf-life of the infused oil is considerably shorter.

Fill a clean, wide-mouth glass jar ⅔ to ¾ full of herb

Pour carrier oil, such as olive oil, over plant material the place lid tightly on jar

___

[38] Criswell, Brooke. "Making Lemon Balm Bundles." *YouTube*, BeWell Bohemia Herbs and Things, June 2019, www.youtube.com/watch?v=50pKk8ExaV4&t=17s.

Set on the counter (some folks say in a sunny window, others
say a dark spot - experiment and choose your preference)
Shake daily to mix oil and herb
Allow to sit for at least two and up to five weeks
Strain and store in a cool, dark, dry place

Penelope Ody, in The Complete Medicinal Herbal, suggests
applying a warmed lemon balm infused oil as an ointment on
chest to help open airways and soothe tension.[39]

As an insect repellent[40]
Rub crushed lemon balm leaves onto a table to thwart insects
Toss a bundle of lemon balm leaves onto a campfire; the smoke
repels insects

As a steam
Place crushed lemon balm leaves into a bowl
Pour boiling water over leaves
Make a loose tent using a towel over the shoulders and head
Breath in steam* be careful, it is steam - hot, moist air - do not
burn yourself, keep a safe distance between you and the bowl,
remove head from tent if the air is too hot
A lemon balm steam reportedly cleanses pores and the skin.

---

[39] Â Ody, Penelope. The Complete Medicinal Herbal. Dorling Kindersley, 1993.

[40] Kowalchik, Claire, and William H. Hylton. Rodale's Illustrated Encyclopedia of Herbs:
Editors. Rodale Press, 1987.

As a recipe item

In Recipes suggests Rodale's Illustrated Encyclopedia

Chop fresh lemon balm leaves and add to orange marmalade

Stuff fresh lemon balm sprigs into a whole fish before grilling or baking; remove sprigs before eating the fish

As a tea

Infuse the lemon balm, fresh or dried, in boiling water to extract many of the beneficial constituents.

1. Boil water

2. Place 2 tsp of fresh or 1 tsp of dried herb per 8 oz water into teapot, press, thermos, or mason jar *The Complete Medicinal Herbal by Penelope Ody states that the infusion is best made from fresh plant material. (aren't you glad you have it growing in your garden?)

3. Pour boiling water over blooms

4. Cover (this is very important, for if uncovered the constituents will rise with the steam, and you will have a less flavorful, less potent cup of tea)

5. Allow to steep for 10 minutes

6. Strain and Enjoy!

Lemon balm flavor can be mild, so blending it with other herbs makes an excellent choice.

The "Medicine Chest" column of the Summer 2017 issue of Herb Quarterly suggests pairing tulsi and lemon balm. "Holy basil [another name for tulsi] and lemon balm blend calms the nerves and uplifts the spirits."[41]

Lemon balm also makes an excellent sun-tea on a hot day. Just clip some stems from a plant, place in lidded glass jar with water, then leave sit in the sun for a few hours to steep.

Another excellent lemon balm beverage is made by placing a few stems in a pitcher with water, and chilling in the fridge for 30 minutes to and hour. Pour a glass a feel how refreshing a beverage lemon balm is.

Cautions/Considerations

Lemon Balm may slow or lower thyroid function if taken in high doses.

---

[41] Â Groves, Maria Noel. "Medicine Chest." *Herb Quarterly, 2017, pp. 20 - 22.*

Notes, comments, questions, drawings... a space for you.

Tulsi
Occimum tenuiflorum

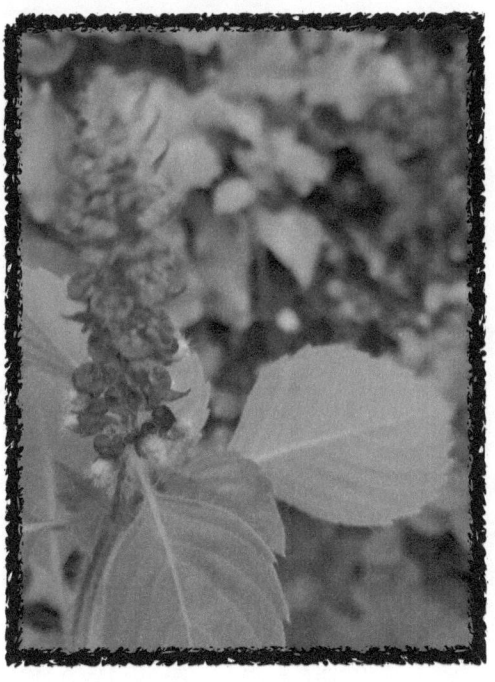

A wonderful plant to befriend, tulsi is easy to grow and offers many physical, psychological and spiritual benefits to the people in its life. Tulsi has a long history as a beloved and sacred plant. Growing a tulsi plant at your home is said to be auspicious. Read on to learn more about this terrific tulsi, and then grow and plant at home.

Tulsi, also frequently called holy basil, has a few closely related species including Ocimum tenuiflorum, O. Americanum Var. Pilosum, O. africanum, and O. gratissimum with similar growing conditions and attributes. I grow, and therefore concentrate my discussion on Occimum tenuiflorum. Tulsi may not be especially well known in contemporary, mainstream American culture; in India, however, tulsi is considered a sacred plant, even the soil beneath a tulsi plant is considered sacred. [42]The plant thus earned the common name 'holy basil'. Folks who revere tulsi as a sacred plant often grow a plant near an entrance or in a central terrace of the home. The plant provides the home, the family, with goodwill, protection, and a connection to the divine. "For every Hindu, keeping a tulsi plant at home is an auspicious thing. Tulsi is believed to promote longevity, positivity and harmony. As per Vastu, placing the tulsi plant near your main door helps to fight negativity and ill-will in the house."[43]

Tulsi, a member of the mint (Lamiaceae) family, charms with gentle purple blooms, soft green leaves, and a soothing, crisp, slightly spicy scent. Though tropical in origin, tulsi grows well in temperate climes as an annual. Tulsi can live as a houseplant through the winter if given a sunny spot. Two potted tulsi plants lived last winter in my laundry room window in the south-east facing corner of the house. The plants more than survived, they bloomed and set seed over the winter months. Tulsi's delicate purple flower is a friend to bees, and many a summer pollinator. The delightful scent rises on the warm

---

[42] Baines, Heather. "The Sacred Benefits of Growing Tulsi." *The Ayurveda Experience Blog,* 25 June 2019, www.theayurvedaexperience.com/blog/the-sacred-benefits-of-growing-tulsi/.

[43] Makaaniq. "Home Sutra: Know The Many Benefits Of Placing A Tulsi Plant At Home." *Home Sutra: Know The Many Benefits Of Placing A Tulsi Plant At Home,* 27 Dec. 2016, www.makaan.com/iq/video/home-sutra-know-the-many-benefits-of-placing-a-tulsi-plant-at-home-video.

summer air. Even the leaves release the spicy sweet aroma. The scent of the tulsi plant is distinct, lovely, sweet, and pungent. Brushing or crushing the leaves releases the scents, and on warm windy days the aroma is carried on the wind. I find breathing the scent calming and soothing. Of a sunny summer day I love to pluck a few tulsi leaves and flowering tops, steep them in freshly boiled water. The resulting tisane provides an enlivening, yet relaxing tea. I find having my own plant the best way to enjoy the brew. I am not a fan of the tulsi tea sold as tea bags in a box from the grocers shelf. However I thoroughly enjoy a cup made from the fresh or dried leaves from a tulsi plant I tended with care and appreciation. The plant makes a delicious tea, both when hot and when cold.

If you have a plant in your garden or in a pot near your door, simply pick some leaves to make a fresh brew. In the high summer, a sun tea of tulsi is a pleasure. Once it is steeped, drink it warm or over ice.

Tulsi will bloom throughout the summer, especially if the blooms are regularly harvested. I have many beds of tulsi throughout the yarden. Many I harvest to dry herb for use later in the year. Others I leave for the pollinators to feed. Eventually I harvest many seeds to start new plants new winter in the greenhouse. Still other stalks I leave standing in the plant to reseed the bed and to feed the wildlife.

A revered plant in India, and renowned for it medicinal properties tulsi deserves to be a recognized and admired. I know I value the beauty, grace, and bounty of the sacred tulsi plant.

Grow, tend, and garden befriend

Growing Conditions: Tulsi originates from India, so you can understand why it likes heat and sun. If you start seeds at home or buy a young tulsi plant start, be sure to await transplanting until after the last frost date. Also, if you are direct sowing seeds, wait until after threat of frost has passed and the soil temperature is warm consistently. Tulsi grows best after the soil is 70 degrees Fahrenheit.

Tulsi will thrive in a sunny spot and a warm location. Tulsi can be grown in a garden bed or container. Bank a host of tulsi plants together, or intersperse tulsi plants amidst vegetables to draw pollinators.

Place a tulsi planter near your door to draw upon the affinity of the plant: "placing the tulsi plant near your main door helps to fight negativity and ill-will in the house."[44] Even if you are not a practitioner of Hindu faith, tulsi can provide spiritual wellness through the act of growing and tending the plant. "Cultivation of tulsi plants has both spiritual and practical significance that connects the grower to the creative powers of nature," notes one study of tulsi published in the scientific Journal of Ayervedic

---

[44] Makaaniq. â€œHome Sutra: Know The Many Benefits Of Placing A Tulsi Plant At Home.â€Â *Home Sutra: Know The Many Benefits Of Placing A Tulsi Plant At Home*, 27 Dec. 2016, www.makaan.com/iq/video/home-sutra-know-the-many-benefits-of-placing-a-tulsi-plant-at-home-video.

<u>and Integrative Medicine</u>.[45] Since wellness comprises spiritual elements, and gardening involves movement, and tulsi supports many body systems, growing tulsi supports well being in a multitude of capacities.

Preferences:
Full sun
Warm soil
Enjoys humid conditions
Thrives in a hot climate

Plant details:
Tulsi plants grow in relation to their environment. If they remain planted in a small container, the plant will stay small. If you plant them in a larger container they will grow larger. Planted in the ground with access to many hours sunlight, adequate water, and with warm temperatures they can reach nearly 2 feet tall when the flower stem emerges. I have plants of varying height and color even though they all sprouted from the same seed pack planted at the same time. Some I never had chance to transplant from the seed tray, they are still alive and blooming, even though each plant is only a few inches tall and a bright yellow-green leaf. I have others planted in 6 inch plastic pots that have reaches 10 - 12 inches tall and are deep green hue of

---

[45] Cohen, Marc Maurice. â€œTulsi - Ocimum Sanctum: A Herb for All Reasons.â€ *Journal of Ayurveda and Integrative Medicine*, Medknow Publications & Media Pvt Ltd, 2014, www.ncbi.nlm.nih.gov/pmc/articles/PMC4296439/.

leaf. I have still more planted in the ground that have medium to dark green leaves and reach 18 inches tall. All these varied plant growth habits attest to the influence of environment on plant growth.

Tulsi flowers abundantly throughout the summer, and as such is a boon to bees and pollinators. The small purple flowers bloom along a single stalk that reaches above the height of the plant leaves. Bloom stems can reach 8 inches tall on a large plant.

If you consistently harvest the flowers, the tulsi will continue to develop new blooms.

Companion Planting Affiliation: Tulsi blooms draw pollinators to the garden benefiting other plants present. Tulsi is said to enhance the success of tomato and potato plants by repelling insects that prey on those nightshade family plants.[46]

Care notes:

Strictly Medicinal Seeds, a nursery specializing in herbal and vegetables seeds and plants, advises "do not overwater [tulsi], and make sure there is good air exchange to keep the plant healthy. Space plants 2 feet apart."[47] The spacing affords room for the plant to bush. When you pinch back tulsi tips, it sends out two new stems. Early pinching of the tulsi plant promotes

---

[46] Wathen, Grace. "Holy Basil Companion Plants." *Garden Guides*, 12 Mar. 2019, www.gardenguides.com/12623382-holy-basil-companion-plants.html.

[47] "Tulsi, Krishna - Holy Basil, Shyama Tulasi (Ocimum Tenuiflorum) Potted Plant, Organic." *Strictly Medicinal Seeds*, 12 Apr. 2019, strictlymedicinalseeds.com/product/tulsi-krishna-holy-basil-shyama-tulasi-ocimum-tenuiflorum-potted-plant-organic/.

bushy plants, and an abundant harvest.

Tulsi may be grown successfully in the container, though unless the container is of sufficient size the growth will be limited to pot size. When in a pot, be sure to water sufficiently without over-watering - allow soil to dry to the touch between waterings. If you have a tulsi in a pot, you may overwinter in a bright spot in doors. I have.

Ways the plants support wellness

In addition to tulsi's beauty in the garden, it offers much to the body. With a long history of use in Ayurvedic practice, tulsi is now gaining awareness and popularity in America. As people learn about the many benefits of tulsi, they are willing to try the tea made from the tulsi plant. Bagged or boxed tulsi tea can even be found in the tea displays at mainstream grocery stores. Among the ways tulsi acts on the body is fostering a decrease of inflammation response, which can be helpful to address the chronic pain associated with inflammation. Tulsi also strengthens digestion and supports blood sugar regulation, explains herbalist Maria Noel Groves in her book <u>Body into Balance.</u>[48]

Scientific study bears out the many attributes of tulsi, according to a 2013 article published in <u>Nutr Cancer,</u> a peer-reviewed medical journal covering research on the role of nutritional

---

[48]Groves, Maria Noel. *Body Into Balance: An Herbal Guide to Holistic Self-Care.* Storey Publishing, 2016.

factors in causing or preventing cancer. The article states, "[Tulsi] possesses anti-inflammatory, analgesic, antipyretic, anti-diabetic, hepatoprotective, hypolipidemic, antistress, and immunomodulatory activities."[49]

You may be thinking, 'I am not versed in these medical terms, what is the list saying?" In a word the list says that tulsi is *great*, or more specifically, in addition to mitigating the inflammation process, tulsi has pain relieving, fever reducing, blood sugar regulating, liver protecting, lipid (fat) regulating, stress mitigating, immune modulating activities.

Obviously, the effects of tulsi are influenced by the tissue state in the body and constitution of the individual, among other factors. Nonetheless, tulsi exerts measurable impact on a variety of body systems. When I refer to tissue state, I mean the current condition of tissue in the body. Constitution refers to an individual's general tendency. If a person has a slow metabolism, they might run cool. If a person is often sedentary or has a tendency for lymph to be stagnant, then they may be 'moist' in constitution because fluid in the cells and lymph stagnates in place rather than moving through the lymph system and into the kidneys for eventual removal or recycling into useful materials. All this is to acknowledge that every person's body is different, and each person is also variable depending on external and internal factors. The aspects of what results from plants, like tulsi, interacting with the individual are influenced by the person's general tendencies (constitution) and

---

[49]Baliga, Manjeshwar Shrinath, et al. "Ocimum SanctumL (Holy Basil or Tulsi) and Its Phytochemicals in the Prevention and Treatment of Cancer." *Nutrition and Cancer*, vol. 65, no. sup1, 2013, pp. 26–35., doi:10.1080/01635581.2013.785010.

the particular moment how they feel (tissue state). The more you become aware of the nuances of your well-being, the more you can notice how you are affected by teas, foods, moods, surroundings…. All the things.

Adding tulsi to your routine, regimes, and rituals offers abundant value.

The Journal of Ayurvedic and Integrative Medicine article, "Tulsi - Occimum Sanctum: An Herb for All Reasons" notes:

> "There is mounting evidence that tulsi can address physical, chemical, metabolic and psychological stress through a unique combination of pharmacological actions. Tulsi has been found to protect organs and tissues against chemical stress from industrial pollutants and heavy metals, and physical stress from prolonged physical exertion, ischemia, physical restraint and exposure to cold and excessive noise. Tulsi has also been shown to counter metabolic stress through normalization of blood glucose, blood pressure and lipid levels, and psychological stress through positive effects on memory and cognitive function and through its anxiolytic and anti-depressant properties."[50]

The same article later explains how tulsi helps combat oxidate stress in the cells by "increasing the body's levels of anti-oxidant

---

[50] Cohen, Marc Maurice. "Tulsi - Ocimum Sanctum: A Herb for All Reasons." *Journal of Ayurveda and Integrative Medicine*, Medknow Publications & Media Pvt Ltd, 2014, www.ncbi.nlm.nih.gov/pmc/articles/PMC4296439/.

molecules such as glutathione and enhancing the activity of anti-oxidant enzymes such as superoxide dismutase and catalase, which protect cellular organelles and membranes by mopping up damaging free radicals."

Energetics: "Warm & Dry (leaf), Cool & Moist (seed); Pungent, Sweet. Vital Stimulant, Relaxant, Tonic".[51] The Sonoran Plant Profile on the Desert Tortoise website describes tulsi's energetics well. The recipes below in this monograph concentrate on leaf and flower, and the constituents contained therein.

Actions: "Alterative, Analgesic, Antibacterial, Antidepressant, Antifungal, Antiviral, Antimicrobial, Anxiolytic, Cardiotonic, Carminative, Demulcent, Diaphoretic, Expectorant, Immunomodulator, Nervine, Radioprotective"[52]

As a nervine: The tulsi monograph from the HerbRally blog explains the multi-faceted interaction tulsi has with the human nervous system. Tulsi initially acts as stimulating, then "follows with a strong sense of calm and feeling grounded. Tulsi opens the heart and mind and encourages devotion and gratitude. It is also considered to energetically support a space of attachment, that which draws and embraces prosperity."
The Herbal Academy blogs also sings tulsi's praises similarly, lauding tulsi's ability to balance. "In Western herbalism, holy

---

[51] Slatterly, John. "Sonoran Plant Profile: Tulsi-Holy Basil." *DesertTortoiseBotanicals.com*, www.desertortoisebotanicals.com/blogs/news/sonoran-plant-profile-tulsi-holy-basil.

[52] Thompson, Krystal. "Tulsi Monograph." *HerbRally*, www.herbrally.com/monographs/tulsi.

basil is considered an adaptogen, helping the body respond in a measured way to stressors (be they physical or emotional), thus reducing the negative effects of stress on physical and emotional health and providing balance."[53]

HerbRally and Herbal Academy are not alone in recognizing the positive, supportive effects tulsi exerts on the nervous system and mental and emotional well-being, many articles and studies discuss the subject. Tulsi supports the bodies capacity to handle physical, environmental, and psychological stresses, especially when tulsi is enjoyed tonically. The many ways tulsi supports metabolic, psychologic, and physiologic wellness is experienced with regular and persistent tulsi ingestion. Make tulsi a part of your daily rituals to enhance its interaction with your mind-body-spirit.

Parts Used: Leaves and flowers (though any aerial part is useable)

When to Harvest: Tulsi may be harvested any time during growing season, especially while blooming before the flower shifts to setting seed.

Regular top-growth harvesting encourages the tulsi plant to grow bushier, so do so, especially early in the growing season. Harvest by cutting stem tops. You can pinch the stem tops between thumb and finger or use scissors. What you do not use immediately, dry for later (to make tea, for example), or make a tincture of fresh plants. There are various techniques for drying

---

[53]Metzger, Jane. "Creating a Local Materia Medica: Holy Basil." *Herbal Academy*, 10 Jan. 2018, theherbalacademy.com/creating-local-materia-medica-holy-basil/.

herbs. You can lay the plant tips on screens in a well ventilated area out of sunlight. If you dry your herbs this way, keep a few things in mind. The screens will need to be placed so that they are safe from pets getting into them. The screens must have plenty of air circulation through them. You do not want dust or debris to settle on the screen, so chose a location not subject to dust or dirt. Drying on screens takes many days to a couple of weeks, so choose a location that is well suited to long term placement. If the air is humid, drying will take longer. Occasionally check the screens while the plant material is drying. Be sure no leaves are touching, and you may even turn plants to ensure even air flow.

If your area is humid, or you are not sure the pant material will dry without mold growth, then use a food dehydrator to speed the drying process.

Another option, especially in sunny and hot times of the year, is to place the harvested plant material into clean paper bags. Roll the top shut and place the bag on the dashboard or back window of a car. Plant material dries in a day or two with this method. Be sure the plant material is loose in the bag with ample air flow. In other words, don't pack the bag full of plant material, rather put only enough that no stems or leaves (or blooms) are crushing any other stems, or leaves (or blooms). Once dry, to separate stems from leaves, rub the stems on a screen; save shredded leaves in airtight container, compost stems. If you do not yet have a screen, you can use a mesh colander or hand separate materials. If some stems end up in the tulsi jar, it is not harmful.

After the plant material is dry, store in a clean, airtight container out of direct light. Light and moisture both shorten the shelf life of dried herbs. If you have dried and stored the herb well, and without mold or bacterial contamination, the dried herb can last a year. If the scent is strong, the herb is still rich with constituents.

How to Prepare

Preparing tulsi can be as simple as pinching of a plant tip popping it in your mouth. I love to do this while weeding the garden. Such a fresh, spicy pop of flavor. I love to put tulsi leaves and flowers into teas, salads, smoothies…tulsi is versatile.

Like chamomile, tulsi accomplishes so much, so mildly. You can drink it every day to tonically support wellness.

As a cooking spice

Add dried or fresh dishes while cooking, as you would basil
Sprinkle leaves over a salad

As an infused oil

You can infuse olive oil with tulsi, thereby imparting the oil with attributes and flavor of tulsi. Making infused oil is simple in process, though it takes weeks for the result.

For the best results, purchase the highest quality olive oil you are able, and check to be sure it is not diluted with other oils. You can make infused oils with either fresh plant material or dried. However, the high water content in fresh plant material means the resulting oil will have a shorter shelf life. The moisture increases the possibility for contamination by microbes, bacterial or fungal. If you are concerned, use dried tulsi.

Making the infused oil:

1. Cut or crush the herbs before placing in jar so that the amount of plant surface in contact with the oil is increased, and to encourage the constituents to infuse into the oil.

2. Fill a clean mason, or other glass jar, ⅔ full with dried herbs.

3. Pour olive oil to cover plant material.

4. Place a lid on the jar to seal tightly. Place the jar in a space where you will easily access it, because you will shake the jar once daily to encourage the oil mixing with the herbs.

5. Gently shake once daily (though don't be concerned if you miss a day or few)
Be sure the lid secures tightly, and check it each time before shaking, obviously, or you will have an oily mess.

6. Allow the jar of oil and herbs to sit, sealed, for 4 weeks. Some folks advise a dark place, others a sunny window, so make your choice.

7. When the four weeks have passed, strain the herbs by pouring the oil through a fine filter, such as a mesh filter or a coffee filter, or tight weave cheese clothe. Use any filter that allows the oil to pass through but catches any plant material.

8. Use the tulsi infused olive oil as you would olive oil - salad dressing, drizzle, dip for fresh baked bread, or pesto.

As I mentioned, if you use freshly harvested tulsi the water content is much higher and decreases the shelf life of the infused oil and increases the risk of mold growth. You can make infused oil with fresh herbs, just consider making a smaller batch that you can use within a couple weeks. Watch for sign of the oil spoiling or goin rancid.

As a tea

Make a delightful and delicious tea with a sweet and spicy flavor by infusing tulsi leaves and/or flowers in boiling (or nearly boiling) water. The boiled water extracts many of the beneficial constituents.

If you are making a cup or mug of tea, place 1- 2 tablespoons or fresh tulsi or 1 tsp of dried herb in the container. If you are making a pot or large mason jar size infusions, then use the above ratio per 8 oz water. I tend to place a generous tablespoon of dried herb in a teapot, or a handful of fresh plant tips. You can use whatever steep-ware you prefer to make the tea: a press, thermos, teapot, or mason jar. You can even make a teabag by putting the herbs in the center of a coffee filter then tie it with twine.

Experiment with herb quantities to find the flavor you enjoy; use more or less herb material to suit your taste. If using fresh tulsi, be sure to cut it up or crush before adding the boiled water.

Once you have selected your steeping method, place your tulsi into the container then pour just boiled water over herb. Be sure to cover the container. Covering the container is very important, for if uncovered the constituents will rise with the steam, and you will have a less flavorful, less potent cup of tulsi tea. Allow the infusion to steep for five to ten minutes. Similar to quantity, experiment with steep duration to find the spot you enjoy the most. Less than five minutes or so, and you will not have extracted much medicinal properties. Now that the infusion is complete, strain and enjoy! Tulsi tea tastes delightful hot or iced.

Tulsi blends well with many herbs, both in flavor and in action. Making a relaxing and carminative (gas relieving) blend including lemon balm and tulsi that synergistically fosters the following list of impacts, according to a summer 2017 issue of Herb Quarterly article, "Carminative Herbs":

> Calms the nerves
> Uplifts the spirit
> Provides stress support
> Provides deep energy
> Support focus[54]

As an infused water or seltzer

A refreshing delight on a summer day, seltzer or an infused water are served chilled. Follow the recipe from the same "Carminative Herbs" article referenced above to try your hand at a tasty beverage treat.

Steep the herbs in room temperature or cold water - a mason jar with a lid works excellently as the container, but any glass jar

---

[54]Groves, Maria Noel. "Carminative Herbs." Herb Quarterly, 2017, pp. 20–22.

with a lid will do. Depending on the type of drink you want to make, use 1.)Carbonated water for a seltzer, or 2.) Still (flat) water for an infused water. Either way, be sure the container has a lid to hold in flavor, aroma, and constituents as the water is infused

Instructions:

1. Place 1 tsp of dried tulsi leaf and flower (per 8 oz water) into mason jar.

2. Add organic rose petals (up to 1 tsp per 8 oz).

3. Pour cold water over herbs.

4. Place lid on the container and infuse at least 20 minutes.

5. Strain, serve and enjoy.

You can leave the herbs in the water and serve by pouring through a strainer into a glass, or serve from a glass container with spigot, or use a bombilla (a straw with a mesh end).

As Support to yoga or meditation practice

Not only do the Hindi revere and value tulsi, yogiis also have a special regard for tulsi. If you have an interest in yoga, holistically, consider what Prashanti de Jagar had to say about tulsi in an article in LA Yoga Magazine, "Tulsi is one of the most important herbs for yoga practitioners, along with anyone who wants a brighter and more sattvic mind, a stronger expansive heart, greater resilience to all forms of stress, and a sharper and more astute immune system."[55]

Cautions/Considerations: Do not take medicinal doses during pregnancy. Tulsi may affect blood sugar levels, so be watchful if diabetic.

---

[55]Jagar, Prashanti de. "Growing Holy Tulsi." *LA Yoga Magazine - Ayurveda & Health*, 11 Apr. 2013, layoga.com/food-home/herbs-spice/growing-holy-tulsi/.

Notes, comments, questions, drawings… a space for you.

Quick Reference Table of Nervine Herbs

Herb	Interaction with Nervous System	Flavor notes
Catnip	relax agitated digestive system, helps manage stress, calming, mildly relaxes nervous system, supports quality sleep,	'Green' or subtly spicy slightly minty flavor
German Chamomile	Relaxant, also relax agitated digestive system, calms while uplifting, supports quality sleep, anxiety relieving, mild pain-relieving action	Mild, long infusions become bitter
Lavender	Antidepressant, helps alleviate tension, supports quality sleep, anxiety relieving, mild pain relieving action	Strong, use small amount of herb in blend
Tulsi	Decreases inflammation, alleviates stressed emotions, anxiety relieving, helps to alleviate sadness or to navigate heavy emotions,	Pungent, spicy flavor
Lemon Balm (Melissa officinalis)	Calms without sedating, improves mood (and cognition), calms nervous digestion, supports quality sleep, anxiety relieving, mild pain relieving action	Mild lemony flavor
Peppermint (Mentha pipperita)	Stimulating, promotes mental clarity, supports quality sleep,	Strong mint flavor
Rose (Rosa rugosa)	Anxiety relieving, helps to alleviate sadness or to navigate heavy emotions,	Sweet, rose flavor, very mild in tea (not as strong as scent)
Bee Balm	Gentle supports quality sleep	Mildly bitter, 'green' flavor
Valerian	Sedates nervous system, relaxes muscles, relaxes blood vessels, supports quality sleep,	Strong smell, strong flavor
Passionflower	Calming and relaxing, mild sedative action, relieves agitation and irritability, mild pain relieving action, which may help soothe nerve pain, effective for stress management, anxiety relieving,	Bitter flavor, use small amount
Basil	Nervous system tonic (taken regularly helps support nervous system function)	Spicy flavor
Plantain	Moistening, which can soothe nerve cells, nutrient rich	Mild, slightly 'green' flavor
Hops	Relaxant, relax irritated digestive system, excellent nerve tonic, soothes irritated and inflamed nerve cells, moistening, nutrient rich, supports quality sleep,	Bitter, strong so a little quantity of herb is sufficient in a blend
Blue vervain	Restorative, calms while uplifting, anxiety relieving, mild pain relieving action	Strongly bitter, use small quantity in blend
Oat straw	Restorative, helps when experiencing sadness, helps to manage anxiety, high in calcium, which supports nervous system function	Green flavor
Licorice root	Nervous system tonic, supports adrenal function (so helpful to stress response and managing stress),	Strong sweet flavor

Keep in mind,

herbs tend to be mild acting, and often accumulate affect slowly over time, meaning drinking the same blend for days in succession before benefit truly imparts.

Always consider the origin of your plant material. If you grow your own, you know about the life of the plant. I recommend using organic herbs when possible. Source your herbs in a way that supports the health of the global plant population (some herbs are at risk of extinction, so if you use those herbs, source them from reputable companies protecting the future of the species. If the plant is not at risk, I still encourage responsible sourcing that adheres to your personal value system.

Tea Blend Ideas

Method of Measurement:

The following blend ideas use the 'simple' method for measurement. An increment is a 'part' and fractions or multiples of part. When you make the blend you choose the size of the part. For example a part could be a tablespoon or a cup. If you like a blend and want to make a large batch to share, you might use a cup. If, however, you want enough for a single pot of tea, you might use a teaspoon as the part.

For example

> 1 part herb A
> ½ part herb B
> 2 parts herb C
> 1 part herb D

The above recipe would translate to:

> 1 tsp herb A
> ½ tsp herb B
> 2 tsp herb C
> 1 tsp herb D

Alternatively, the same example recipe above, would translate into:

> 1 cup herb A
> ½ cup herb B
> 2 cup herb C
> 1 cup herb D

Using the 'simple' measurement system, I crafted some "Tea of Tranquility" blends.

---

1. Emotional Soothe - a tea to help alleviate or navigate difficult or heavy emotions.

> 1 part chamomile flower
> 1 part catnip leaf
> 1 part rose petals (roses you have grown your self or

organic only! Lots of noxious chemicals are sprayed on commercial roses, do not ingest them.)

> ¼ part lavender flowers

---

2. Balancing Soothe - a tea to center the mind-body-spirit
> 1 part chamomile flower
> 1 part lemon balm leaf
> 1 part catnip leaf
> 1 part tulsi leaf and bloom

---

3. I am ready for bed, but can't fall asleep - a tea to help quiet the mind and promote the transition to sleep
> 1 part passionflower aerial parts
> 1 part chamomile flower
> ½ part valerian root
> ¼ part hops
> ⅛ part blue vervain leaf

---

4. Relax into sleep - a tea relax the nervous and digestive

systems and calm anxiety

    ¼ part lavender flower

    ½ part chamomile flower

    ¼ part mint leaf

    1 part catnip leaf

---

5. Calm, cool, and collected - a tea to quietly stimulate the mind and keep the nerve cells smooth and cool

    1 part tulsi leaf and bloom

    1 part plantain leaf

    1/4 to 1/2 part peppermint leaf

---

6. Steady as she goes - a centering blend that supports emotional well-being, peace of mind, and supports facing the next phase of the days activities

    2 parts tulsi

    1 part chamomile

    1 part catnip

    1 part lavender

    1 part rose petals (roses you have grown your self or organic only! Lots of noxious chemicals are sprayed on commercial roses, do not ingest them.)

---

7. Tummy calm - a tea to soothe an agitated digestive system

with some tasty support

    1 part catnip leaf

    1 part chamomile flower

    1 part tulsi leaf and bloom

    1 part fennel seed

    ¼ part hops

---

8. Cool as a cucumber - a cooling, calming, moistening blend, excellent iced on a hot day.

    3 parts lemon balm leaf

    1 part tulsi leaf and bloom

    1 part plantain leaf

    1/4 to 1/2 part peppermint leaf

Infusion Instructions; or how to make herbal tea:

When you make tea with herb leaves or flowers, if you use fresh you will always need more plant material to get the flavor and medicinal constituents, because fresh plant leaf and bloom are comprised of mostly water. Dried herb is much more concentrated, so less plant material yields the same or greater flavor and medicinal constituent content.

To make the tea:

1. Heat the water. I like my tea piping hot, so I use water a a rolling boil, others prefer to use water that is just about to boil. Trust your preference.

2. While the water boils, prepare your steep ware. There are many ways you can make loose leaf tea. You can use a ceramic or porcelain teapot, you can use a glass French press, you can use a tea ball, or you can use a cloth teabag…. Find a system that is comfortable for you.

3. Place, per 8 oz water , 1 tablespoon of fresh or 1 teaspoon of dried herb leaf or flower into teapot, press, thermos, or mason jar

4. Pour boiling water over the plant material in the steep-ware.

5. Cover! This is very important, for if uncovered the constituents will rise with the steam, and you will have a less flavorful, less potent cup of tea. If your chosen steep-ware has a lid, like a tea pot or French press, then this is easy to accomplish. If, however, you are using a mug, find a saucer to set atop the mug while your tea steeps. If you are using a mason jar, screw the lid on loosely, so it is not vacuum tight when you try to open it in a few minutes. You are resourceful, if your steep-ware is

lidless, you will think of a solution.

6. Allow to steep for 10 minutes. The long steep time infuses the medicinal properties into the water. You can steep the tea for less time if you prefer a mild tasting tea; however, know that it will have little medical properties. You can allow the tea to steep longer, for a stronger tea, too. Experiment and note your preferences regarding flavor, texture (some herbs have a smooth feel, a syrupy texture after prolonged steep - try soaking a broken cinnamon stick in a glass mason jar full of water overnight, and you will see what I mean), and effects on body, mood, and energy, T. Find what you like.

7. Strain and Enjoy!

Some steep-ware make preparing the tea a breeze. A French press, for example, you push down the plunger and pour, voila - strained tea. Others types of steep-ware require the use of a tea strainer (or any strainer, really). You pour the tea through the strainer into the cup to remove bits of leave, or other plant material. Some teapots have a strainer built-in on the inside where the spigot connects to the body of the teapot, others do not, so take a look before you fill the teapot.

Making tea can be a ritual. The very act of preparing the material, awaiting the boil, handling the steep-ware, and awaiting the infusion can be intention, can be part of finding and experiencing tranquility. The process or preparing the materials and making the tea allows you to slow down and be fully present for a moment. That is a gift. Then when you hold the warm cup in your hand, breath in the aroma, that is another moment building the tranquility. Then the tea itself. Ah. What a wonderful act. A cup of tea.

Share a pot of catnip tea, and expand the effect to community. A simple cup of tea addresses many aspects of wellness. The herb nourishes the body and supports body system function, the ritual of making tea attends spirituality, sharing tea forges connections with others. A pot of tea is an excellent instance of the multi-faceted nature of wellness, and the power of healing inherent in forming personal relationships with plants.

Of course, you can also make teas as a hot infusion, then cool in the refrigerator and drink them as an iced-tea. Or, make them as a sun tea. Put the herbs, fresh harvested or dried, into a clear glass jar with a tight fitting lid. Then set it in a sunny sport for a few hours. Strain and drink sun-dappled warm, or pour over ice.

Another refreshing way to enjoy tea of tranquility in summer is to brew the blend, then freeze 1/2 the tea into ice-cube, and chill 1/2 the tea. Once the cubes have frozen, fill a glass with cubes of tea, pour chilled tea over, and if you are feeling fancy, add a sprig of fresh herb to the glass, then enjoy the fruits of your herbal tea blending adventure.

You can grow and harvest your own herbs, and have a yarden adventure crafting your own herbal wonders.

Glossary

Action: the impact an herb has on the body, or the way an herbal constituent or herb interacts with the body

Adaptogen: helps the body manage the stress response

Aerial parts: all parts of the plant that grow above ground: leaves, stems, and flowers

Analgesic: pain relieving

Antidepressant: Alleviates depression to a system, through various mechanisms

Anti-inflammatory: reduces inflammation in the body through various mechanisms depending on the specific herb and the specific tissue involved.

Anti-microbial: Resistent to microbes. Some herbs or constituents react to a wide range of pathogens, while others have a specific target. Investigate the specific herb or phytochemical to learn more about what / which microbes it is effective against.

Anti-Oxidant: helps prevent oxidative stress to the body.

Anti-septic: stops or slows the growth of micro-organisms

Anti-spasmodic: prevents, stops, or reduces the spasming of muscle tissue, smooth or skeletal-muscular

Anxiolytic: reducing anxiety. Often subtle in effect, and require long term (tonic) exposure. Some herbs act more acutely, but none have the intensity associated with pharmaceutical anxiety medication

Antipyretic: fever reducing. There are various ways an herb or herbal constituent can interact with the body to reduce fever; it could do with circulation, or pore dilation, or other specifics.

Aromatic: refers to plants constituents that have particular molecular structure, and release a strong aroma when those molecules are damaged.

Aroma Therapy: treatment or action that is catalyzed by scent; the use of scent to alter mood, or influence the nervous system

Bitter: A flavor that stimulates the digestive juices. A flavor, that is sharp and often considered 'unpleasant', yet it indicates to the digestive system to get the digestive juices flowing, thereby supporting digestive system function

Blend: to combine various herbs to create a synergistic result

Carminative: Relieves gas in the digestive system

Cholagogue: Supports bile flow, which supports digestion and detoxification

Constituent: chemical compounds within a plant; the pars of the plant chemical structure that generate effect

Constitution: refers to a person's natural tendency regarding energetics. For example, some folks tend to be 'dry' while others tend to be 'moist'; some folks tend to be warm, while others tend to be cool. Individuals do experience tissue states at variance with their constitution due to various factor, such as injury, illness, fatigue or many others. Learning to recognize a persons constitution helps to select an herb well-suited for the individual and situation.

Diaphoretic: promotes sweating

Decoct: to simmer plant material in water over a long period of time. Barks, roots, and seeds, the hard and dry parts of plants, tend to need to be decocted in order to extract their qualities. Some plant constituents require very long decoctions indeed in order to extract, like the complex carbohydrates in medicinal mushrooms.

Diuretic: promotes urination, or the movement of waste water from cells to urine

Emmenagogue: stimulates mensus, or contraction of the uterus

Energetics: the manner in which plant tends to impact human tissue; a set of ranges, wet/dry; lax/tense; hot/cold

Hepatoprotective: action that protects the liver

Herb: a plant used for medicinal properties, or as a spice or culinary item

Herbal Energetics: A reference system discussing tissue states and herbal actions on the body.   The system relies on a series of continuums, hot / cold, tense / lax, dry / moist. Learning to recognize the persons tissue state helps to choose an herb to mitigate, or balance that state. If someone is 'hot' (after mowing the grass on a hot day, for example) then a 'cooling' herb (like watermelon) helps to cool down the person's tissue state.

Holistic: a science, practice, or philosophy that is characterized by a consideration of a multitude of parts comprising a whole; in the context of health, wellness, and personal care, holistic refers to the treatment of the whole person, taking into account mental, emotional, social and environmental factors, rather than just the symptoms of a disease.

Hypnotic: help to promote or sustain deep sleep. Hypnotic herbs interact with the nervous system in a way that supports deep and restful sleep. Some are mild or gentle, whereas others have a stronger more immediate impact. Be sure to explore the intensity of the hypnotic effect and impact on your constitution so you know how your body will react.

Immunomodulatory: modulate immune function. This means, the herb or herbal constituent helps bring immune function into balance. If an immune system is sluggish or under-active, then the herb helps activate immune function; if however, the immune system is over-active, as in an auto-immune disorder, then the herb helps calm the immune system.

Infuse: "to steep or soak (leaves, bark, roots, etc.) in a liquid so as to extract the soluble properties or ingredients." [source: Dictionary.com] For example, making a cup of tea is an infusion. In the case of a cup of tea, water is the solvent, and the plant material, black tea, in a tea bag is placed in the hot water. As the tea steeps, the flavor and plant constituents are extracted into the water, resulting in a change in color (from clear to brown) and flavor. When you make an infusion using herbs, the same process occurs.

Nervine: any constituent or herb that has an effect on the nervous system, whether relaxing or stimulating

Phytochemicals: the molecules, elements, and chemical compounds found in the plant; often identified and discussed in researching or explaining the hows and whys of plant effect on human physiology

Refrigerant: promotes cooling of the tissue

Sedative: Lowers the activity of a system, often the digestive system   .

Stimulant: activate or increase body system function; stimulate activity

Synergistic: When the combined effect is greater than the sum of the individual effect. (if you are a Harry Potter fan think like Hermione when she stated Golpalott's Third Law,""*The antidote for a blended poison will be equal to more than the sum of the antidotes for each of the separate components.*")[56]

Tissue state: the condition, temporary or longer lasting, that a tissue is in. For example, if you have had lots of salt and your body is retaining water, then the tissue state of the portion of the body retaining water is 'moist'.

Tonic: refers to an herb that may be taken at medicinal doses daily over an extended period of time; tonic also refers to an herb that has a sustaining support impact on a tissue or system.

---

[56] Rowling, Joanne K. Harry Potter and the Half-Blood Prince. Bloomsbury, 2014.

Volatile Oil: plant constituents that easily evaporate at normal temperatures, that are extracted and concentrated, usually through distillation. Also called essential oils. *think essence for essential, and volatile, as in easily evaporated

Thanks for reading, and I hope you enjoyed the book.

Visit my website to learn more about herbs

https://bewellbohemiaherbsandthings.blogspot.com

Visit my online store to find plants, seeds, steep-ware, and information about workshops and BeWell Bundles

https://bewell-bohemia-herbs-and-things.square.site/s/shop

BeWell

You deserve to.